By Christopher Dow

Fiction
Effigy
    Book I: Stroud
    Book II: Oakdale
The Books of Bob
    Devil of a Time
    Jumping Jehovah
The Clay Guthrie Mysteries
    The Dead Detective
    Landscape with Beast
    The Texas Troll Express
Roadkill
The Werewolf and Tide, and Other Compulsions

Nonfiction
Lord of the Loincloth (nonfiction novel)
The Wellspring: An Inquiry into the Nature of Chi
Circling the Square: Observations on the Dynamics of Tai Chi Chuan
Elements of Power: Essays on the Art and Practice of Tai Chi Chuan
Alchemy of Breath: An Introduction to Chi Kung
Book of Curiosities: Adventures in the Paranormal
Living the Story: The Meandering, Wonderful, and True Adventures of
    an Unknown Writer
    Vol.I: Growing Up Takes Time
    Vol. II: Growing Old Takes Longer

Poetry
City of Dreams
The Trip Out
Texas White Line Fever
Networks
Puzzle Pieces: Selected Poems

Editor
The Abby Stone: The Poetry of Bartholo Dias
The Best of Phosphene
The Best of Dialog

Elements of Power

Elements of Power

Essays on the Art and Practice of Tai Chi Chuan

Christopher Dow

Phosphene Publishing Company
Temple, Texas

Elements of Power: Essays on the Art and Practice of Tai Chi Chuan
© 2017/2021 by Christopher Dow
ISBN 13: 978-0-9986316-4-6

Published by Phosphene Publishing Company
Temple, Texas, U.S.A.
phosphenepublishing.com

2.1-3/21

Dedicated to you, dear Tai Chi lover.

Contents

Elements of Power

Introduction

What exactly is Tai Chi Chuan?

We can say that it is an effective martial art and a healthful exercise, but we also have to admit that it is an art born of mystery since we don't really know who invented it. Was it created by the legendary Taoist monk Chang San-feng, the Chen family of Henan Province, or someone between, such as itinerate martial artist Wang Tsung-yueh, who reputedly taught the Chens? We'll probably never know, and this adds to the art's mystique, lending Tai Chi a sense of emerging directly from the Tao as a gift to humankind.

We also can say that it is an art of contradictions. You move slowly in order to be able to move fast. You move deliberately in order to be able to move spontaneously. You move with continuity so that you can disrupt continuity in others. You separate solidness and emptiness only to recombine them. You strive to be like steel embedded in cotton.

Obviously, Tai Chi is not a particular form or specific set of movements, otherwise there would be only one version instead of the variety we now see: five major recognized styles and numerous modified, abbreviated, or hybrid forms. But the efficacy of these many styles—several of which are very different in appearance, "flavor," and even specific points of utility—indicates that each has qualities that define it as an art that can be called "Tai Chi."

In this book, we will explore what "Tai Chi" means, but this is not a thorough exegesis of Tai Chi. That's already been done better by others. Nor is it intended to explicate particular aspects of form or martial usage, per se. Those aspects also have received expert treatment in the hands of others. Instead, this book is a collection of essays, many of which I wrote to help explain Tai Chi matters to my students. Others are what might be called gee-whiz essays that were sparked by a passage in my book, *Circling the Square: Observations on the Dynamics of Tai Chi Chuan*. In that passage, I noted the very real and significant similarities between the Microcosmic Orbit of chi circulation within the human body and the physical and energetic structure of the electrostatic generator known as the Van de Graaff generator. Once I noticed this similarity, it opened me to a great number of other congruencies between various aspects of Tai Chi and objects, mechanical systems, energy constructs, and ideas. The more I delved into these similarities, the more of them I noticed, and they excited me enough to want to write about them.

And now for the caveat. The essays in this volume were written as independent pieces over a period of time, and when I wrote them, I wasn't thinking about collecting them together into a volume. Once I did collect them, though, I realized that I probably should apologized in advance for any replication of material that can be found in my other books on Tai Chi and chi kung. While these essays demonstrate—I hope—the great diversity of Tai Chi's relationships with the practitioner and the world at large, the art has a somewhat focused range of activities and principles. This means that any writer on the subject will keep returning to those actions and precepts. Because of that, anyone who writes enough about Tai Chi will naturally go over familiar ground even in the midst of explaining novel ideas. After all, one frequently repeats Tai Chi movements, such as Single Whip or Brush Knee Twist Step, when doing the form, even while one is discovering new functions for them.

In all cases, my self-plagiarism was in the service of the topic of the essay. Often, I found that what I'd written elsewhere expressed the ideas about as well as I could, and there seemed to be little point in either paraphrasing myself or trying to do a rewrite that would essentially say the same thing but more poorly. However, I've only included essays here in which the borrowings are nil or comprise but a limited portion of the whole, and I've left out essays that are basically extensive rewrites of material that has previously appeared in my other books, even if they do contain some new material.

Likewise, please forgive the occasional repetition of illustrations. Because these essays sometimes track over similar ground, they also require the same illustrations. So please accept my apologies in advance for these replications. They are not, I assure you, extensive. It also should be noted that when you see illustrations with multiple images representing an animation, you should go to the appropriate Internet link mentioned in the "Notes" appendix, where you can see the animation in action. Most of these are both fun and instructive.

The reader might wonder why I capitalize Tai Chi when referring to the art, but lower case the words when referring to the tai chi symbol. The art is, I feel, an entity in its own right—a proper noun. We can talk about karate and kung fu in the lower case because those words represent not simply a range of different styles but an equally diverse range of principles. They are generic terms. Various Tai Chi styles, on the other hand, differ mainly in their specific methods, but the principles of Tai Chi support the foundations of all of them. Tai Chi is a unified art with many expressions, while kung fu, for example, represents a diversity of arts with different expressions. I refer to other specific martial styles also in the upper case, such as Shaolin Long Fist or Hapkido.

Even though my intention with this book isn't to explain the Tai Chi form, its martial usage, or any specific health aspects the form promotes, my hope is that these essays will further and deepen your practice of Tai Chi no matter what style you pursue or your intentions in pursuing it. The simple fact is that Tai Chi principles and dynamics can be found in many and sundry places in the world, and the reason for that is the naturalness of the art. We only have to open our eyes, minds, and bodies to find that naturalness within ourselves as well as within the world.

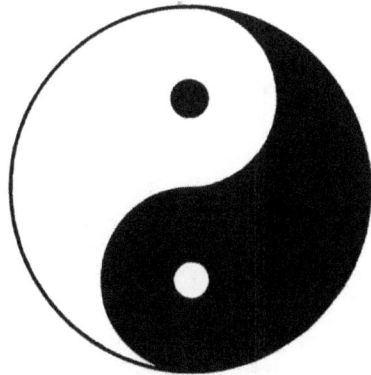

Part I

Roots

1. A Historical and Personal Perspective on Tai Chi Chuan

To understand the origins of Tai Chi Chuan, and all Oriental martial arts, we must go back nearly 5,000 years in Chinese history. In the twenty-seventh century BC, two courses of events began that pioneered what the world now thinks of as kung fu. First, primitive stylized forms of personal combat began to arise. A weapons form was devised by the legendary Yellow Emperor of China, Huang Ti, who won an important military victory using this early martial art. About a hundred years later, the cruel warlord Chi-Yu invented go-ti, a bloody sport in which the combatants donned helmets armed with horns and attempted to gore each other. At about the same time, the second course took an entirely different approach to physical culture. Scholar-monks began to develop series of medical gymnastics coupled with respiratory techniques, called chi kung (chi gong).

Martial techniques continued to evolve, as did the depth and breadth of chi kung. Confucius, in the fifth century BC, mentioned the need for military arts among the six arts he taught his disciples. And the Taoist writings of Lao Tzu, an older contemporary of Confucius, had a profound influence on the development of kung fu in general and on chi kung in particular by emphasizing nonresistance to the natural order as well as self-development. The Taoists further developed respiratory techniques and the psycho-physiological emphasis so important to chi kung.

The parallel courses of kung fu and chi kung continued until the sixth century, when, so it said, a visitor from India took up residence at the Shaolin temple in Honan province. He was Ta-Mo, the son of a Brahman king, also called

Bodhidharma, or Master. (Figure 1.1) His teachings radically altered not only the practices of the monks of the Shaolin temple but ultimately the entire course of religious and philosophical thought in China, Korea, and Japan.

The Shaolin temple had been built three centuries earlier, and there monks prayed and led ascetic lives. When he first arrived, Ta-Mo noticed that the monks, though devout, were weak, unhealthy, and prone to fall asleep during prayers and meditations due to their acetic lifestyle. He taught them dhyana, or yogic concentration, from his own Buddhist background to aid them in focusing their attention. The Chinese transliterated dhyana to Ch'an. As the practice spread further east to Japan, it came to be called Zen. Ta-Mo also introduced three series of exercises designed to strengthen the monks' bodies. These exercises, called the Change of Tendons, the Marrow Washing, and Eighteen Buddha Hands, formed the roots of Shaolin kung fu.

During the next few centuries, Ta-Mo's exercises combined with two other exercise forms already practiced in China. One of these was a sequence of animal movements devised by the brilliant third-century physician Hua T'o that consisted of jumping, twisting, swaying, crawling, rotation, and contraction. (Figure 1.2) The second was chi kung, the Taoist meditative-respiratory techniques initially practiced for health. The Shaolin temple priests evolved these static exercises and combined them with already existing martial arts to create five mobile forms useful for self-defense.

These five forms were named after animals whose traits they embodied: tiger for strengthening bones and jumping; dragon for attention, spirit, and stillness; leopard for application of force and fighting; snake for inner breathing, sensitivity, and action; and crane for concentration, stability, and accuracy. All were of an external nature, emphasizing physical strength, hardness, and speed. Over the centuries, these five Shaolin forms proliferated into more than four hundred individual styles of kung fu in China, and the techniques spread to other countries to

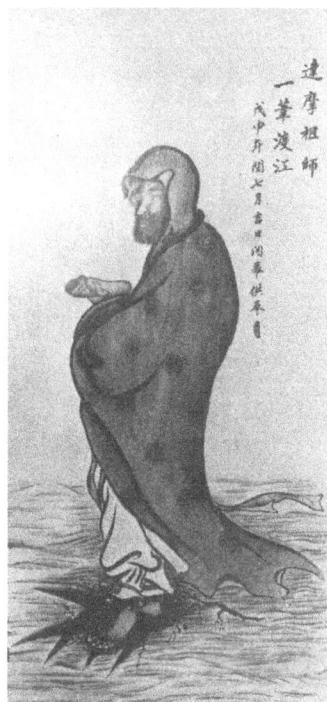

Figure 1.1 Bodhidharma, who introduced the basics of chi kung and kung fu to monks at the Shaolin Temple, rides across the Yellow River on a palm leaf.

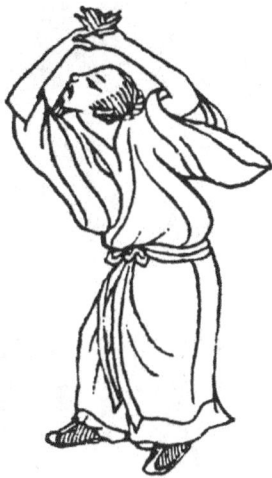

Bird

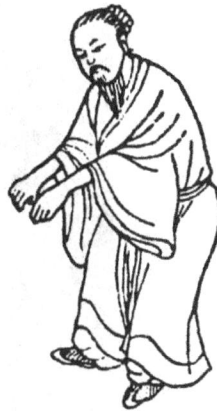

Deer

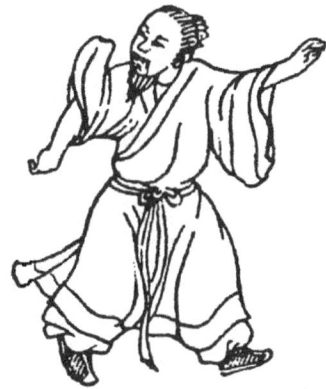

Monkey

Figure 1.2 Hua T'o's Five Animal Frolics were chi- and strength-building exercises based on the movements of animals.

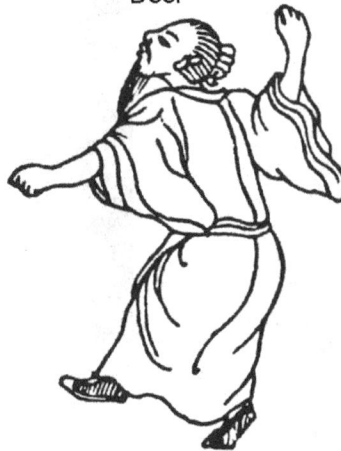

Bear

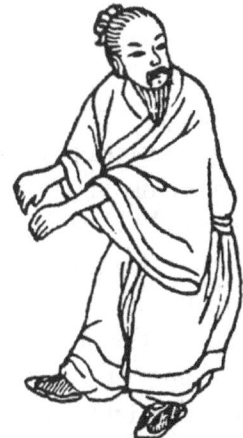

Tiger

make up the basis of Korean Taekwondo, Japanese karate, and scores of other styles of personal combat in Vietnam, Thailand, and elsewhere.

Intermixed in the chronicles of kung fu is the often apocryphal but always entertaining history of Tai Chi Chuan. It all began in the thirteenth century with a Taoist monk named Chang San-feng. (Figure 1.3) Chang had studied Shaolin boxing at the temple and mastered the techniques after ten years, but he became disenchanted with the brute strength and strenuous exertions of the Shaolin forms. He left the temple and wandered until he came to the Wudang Mountains in Hupeh Province. One morning he was awakened by the sounds of a struggle. Hastening to the location, he witnessed a fight between a stork and a snake.

The stork was much larger, stronger, and faster than the snake and struck repeatedly with quick, hard jabs of its beak, but the snake sinuously and softly avoided the blows. The stork often overbalanced as it missed its target, giving the snake opportunity to counterstrike when the stork was most vulnerable. At last the stork fell down, defeated. Chang saw that supple, yielding force could vanquish overpowering and hard superior strength.

That night when he lay down to sleep, Chang was visited in his dreams by Emperor Hsuan Wu the Great. The emperor taught him the rudiments of an internal boxing style that made the body supple and yielding and that dramatically increased its potential for intrinsic energy. Chang practiced his new internal boxing style, and not too long afterwards, he left the mountains. While traveling, he was attacked by a band of brigands, and he soundly defeated them all using his new style, which eventually evolved into Tai Chi Chuan.

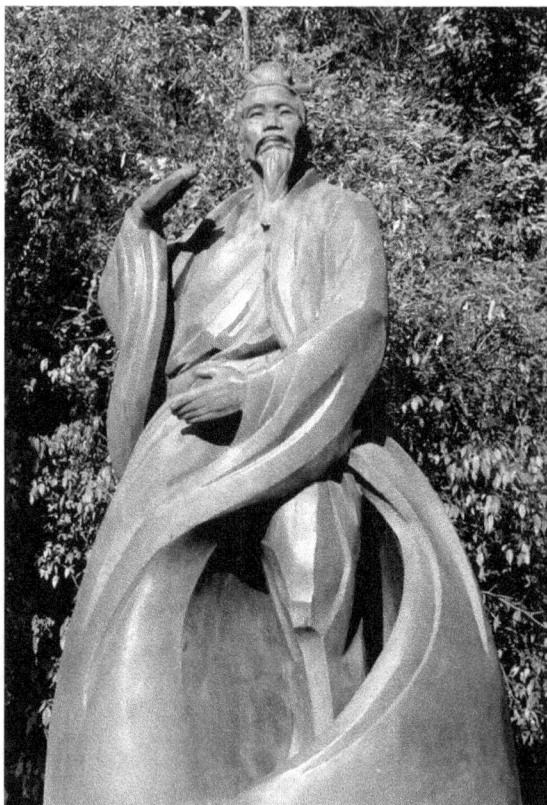

Figure 1.3 A statue of Chang San-feng, the legendary founder of Tai Chi Chuan, in the Wudang Mountains of China, where he supposedly witnessed the battle between a bird and a snake that inspired him to create Tai Chi.[1]

It's a wonderful story and, like much folklore, might have a grain of truth to it. Though the records are few and sketchy, there is historical evidence that Chang actually lived. We even have a date for his birth—April 9, maybe in the year 1247. (See the next chapter for a more apocryphal take on Chang and his exploits.) If indeed he was an actual historical person who played a significant role in the development of Tai Chi, he probably practiced external Shaolin forms and either developed an internal style or integrated various internal elements into one style that was akin to what we now call Tai Chi. However, there is no mention of martial arts, much less Tai Chi, in the records of Chang's life, and the Chen family, from whom we have direct historical lineage of Tai Chi, do not mention Chang in their histories. Not only that, but the earliest historical record to mention Chang's connection to any martial art is in "Epitaph for Wang Zhengnan," written by Huang Zong-xi in 1669.

Like many creators of martial styles, Chang might be apocryphal or even mythical. But mythic or not, we credit him with distinguishing the internal from the external. The external consists of regulation of breath, training of bone and muscle, the ability to advance and retreat, and the unity of hard and soft. The internal consists of training of sinew and muscle, exercise of chi kung, subduing offense by stillness, and defeating an enemy the instant he attacks. On a more basic level, the external is the linkage between eye, fist, and foot, while the internal is the integration of will, vital energy, and internal power. So, while it's unlikely that Chang—mythic or not—invented Tai Chi as we now know it, he is celebrated as the founder of the art.

But, if Chang San-feng didn't create Tai Chi, who did? Again the answer is buried in antiquity, but from the dimness come two major possibilities, both of which involve the Chen family of Henan Province. The first is that Tai Chi was developed by one of two Chen patriarchs. The earlier of these was Chen Pu of the sixteenth century, but his tombstone, inscribed by his tenth-generation lineal descendant, makes no mention of Tai Chi, which it almost certainly would have if he had originated it. The latter was Chen Wang-ting of the seventeenth century, a famous fighter who wrote a treatise on boxing. His book, however, does not specifically mention Tai Chi.

The absence of references to Tai Chi for these two men might not be unusual, however, because the art was initially known simply as Chen family boxing or the Thirteen Postures. The name Tai Chi Chuan was given to the art by Ong Tong-he in the mid 1880s, when he witnessed a demonstration by the great and undefeated Yang Lu-chan. After watching Yang defeat everyone who challenged him, Ong wrote, "Hands holding tai chi shakes the whole world, a chest containing ultimate skills defeats a gathering of heroes."[2] In saying this, he was referring to how the art translated the philosophy of the tai chi symbol into physical movement. (See "Symbolic Movement" and "Natural Patterns," later in this book.) So, it remains historically unclear how the Chens first developed Tai Chi.

The second possibility again smacks of the apocryphal, but it does make sense in light of the Chens' sudden acquisition of Tai Chi. In this version, the true founder of the art is unknown, though it may have been Chang San-feng. In the 19th century, a skilled exponent of internal boxing, one Wang Tsung-yueh, or perhaps Wang's disciple, Chiang Fa, passed through the Chen village.

While there he witnessed the local style and later made disparaging remarks about it. He was promptly challenged by the Chens, whom he soundly and easily defeated. The Chens requested that Wang (or Chiang) stay and teach them, and Wang helped them modify their native boxing, Cannon Fist, to create Chen style Tai Chi. Chen Style, from which all other modern Tai Chi styles are derived, is a vigorous routine, with fast punches and jumps into the air.

This theory is lent further credence by the fact that the people of the nearby village of Zhaobao have their own Tai Chi style that is very similar to Chen Style. And it seems to be just as old and just as mysteriously acquired, though Wang Tsung-yueh does figure in the Zhaobao backstory. So, it is possible that an itinerant martial artist—Wang or Chiang—spent time in both villages during his travels and left his knowledge with the people at both locations, though the Chens deny this, insisting that Zhaobao learned from the Chens. That would make the Zhaobao villagers the first to have acquired Tai Chi from the Chens, which seems unlikely considering the great difficulties encountered by Yang Lu-chan when he approached the Chens for instruction.

The dissemination of Tai Chi outside of the Chen clan began soon after, and that story, too, contains its share of mystery. It begins with Yang Lu-chan, born in 1799. Yang had heard of the Chens' great skill and sought instruction from family expert, Chen Chang-shin. Here the story takes on several versions; in the most commonly told one, Yang was refused instruction because he wasn't a family member. Undaunted, he became a servant and secretly observed training sessions, practiced on his own, and learned. After being discovered practicing, he was personally taught by Chen Chang-shin, who realized Yang's potential. Whatever the truth of the origin of Yang's instruction, he was the first person outside of the Chen clan to be taught the art, though at about the same time Wu Yu-hsiang also learned Chen Style and went on to found his own style, originally called Wu Style, then Old Wu, but now generally referred to as Wu/Hao, or simply as Hao Style because Wu did not have offspring and passed his style to noted expert and Tai Chi Classics contributor Li I-yu, who then taught the Hao family.

After leaving Chen village, Yang moved to Beijing, where he popularized the art. He loved to match skills with other martial artists, and not only was he undefeated, he never seriously injured an opponent. His grandson, Yang Chen-fu, who died in 1936, slowed and expanded the movements and shortened the length of the set to codify the Yang form and is credited with defining and regulating the principles of Yang Tai Chi. One of his disciples, Cheng Man-ching, who died in 1975, reached the highest levels of the art and was one of the earliest practitioners to spread it to the United States.

A major variation of Yang Style is Wu Style (not to be confused with Wu/Hao Style), which traces its origins to Yang Ban-hou, son of Yang founder Yang Lu-chan and uncle of Yang Chen-fu. At the time, Yang Style had three variations of the form: low, middle, and high stances. The movements were basically the same, but the martial expression of each was slightly different. Yang Ban-hou was a fierce fighter who utilized the middle and high stances rather than the low stance, and his movements were more compact and utilized smaller circles. He reputedly was so mean, unpleasant, and brutal that only three students could stand his training regimen. One of them was Quan Yu, a guard for the royal Manchurian household, who changed his surname to Wu. He practiced, essentially, what he learned from Yang Ban-hou, but his son, Wu Chien-chuan, who learned from both his father and Yang Ban-hou, modified the art to create a distinct small-frame form.

This small-frame form was further developed by Chien-Chuan's son, Wu Kung-i. Now, several generations later, Wu is a recognizably different style. Its movements are much more compact than those of Yang Style, and it has a higher stance. Yang and Wu are by far the most popular Tai Chi styles, both in China and the United States, but Chen Style's popularity has been on the rise. There is one other officially recognized major Tai Chi style, Sun Style, created by Sun Lu-tang, which combines Tai Chi with elements of Bagua and Hsing-I, two other internal martial arts. Today, there are many other hybrid styles, but all derive from one of the five major styles: Chen, Wu/Hao, Yang, Wu, and Sun. Each style has its special emphasis and flavor, but all adhere to the basic principles of Tai Chi.

With so many styles, one might ask, "What is Tai Chi?" Certainly Tai Chi embodies physical technique, but the great diversity between styles eliminates physical technique as the primary definer. The chi kung aspect of Tai Chi is at least as important as is martial technique. Tai Chi is a subtle feeling, an awareness, and a pointed concentration. The true techniques of Tai Chi are internal, and you learn them gradually the more you practice. Foremost among them are relaxation, centered awareness, concentrated attention, soft and continuous motion, calmed thought, and a vibrant, energetic inner strength. Herein rests the true beauty of Tai Chi, for although it has roots in a long tradition of martial arts and is proven to be effective in that realm, it has equally deep roots in the healthful practice of chi kung. This is what makes Tai Chi such a well-rounded exercise as well as an excellent martial art. And in our modern, hectic times, the healthful aspects are perhaps more important than the martial applications. After all, few of us will have occasion to fight, but we all could use a formula for enhancing our daily health and well-being and easing the effects of aging.

Tai Chi players come to the art in many ways. We've all heard many things about it: it's a gentle martial art, it's healthful, it's relaxing, it's a non-strenuous but effective exercise, it's so beautiful to watch, it's mystical. Each person is drawn by his or her own reasons. My personal journey along the Tai Chi path began in 1980. I enjoyed keeping fit and had an exercise routine consisting mostly of calisthenics and stretching that I had been happy with for several years. But something was lacking. True, I was strong and flexible because of my workouts, but I felt I wanted more direction, more purpose. I began to look toward the martial arts.

At the time, the worldwide proliferation of martial arts was in its infancy, and like many people at the time, I was aware of the martial arts from a few films and TV shows and a scattering of public demonstrations, but I didn't know much about them. A little research was enough to boggle me. There were literally hundreds of types. Where should I begin? I examined my own needs and compared those with what little I'd learned of the various martial styles. I was turned off by the regimentation, violence, and sport aspects of karate and Taekwondo. That left me with some form of kung fu, or wushu, as some of the more modern Chinese forms are called. The name Tai Chi kept cropping up, and the more I learned about it the better it seemed for me. The only person I knew who actually practiced a martial art was a man who had earned a black belt in karate while stationed in Okinawa in the early 1960s. I asked him what martial art he would recommend, and his immediate reply was, "Tai Chi."

I guess the main factor that really drew me to the art was its longevity. It's an art that improves with age. External styles depend on muscle and bone, which is all well and good for the younger practitioner, but Tai Chi depends on sinew and breath, which can remain powerful even in advanced age. I was nearly thirty, and though I would probably have gotten competent at an external style, it would have been a constant struggle just to maintain my own status quo. If I was going to put that much effort into something, I wanted to be able to get the most out of it. That Tai Chi players reportedly not only maintain proficiency but improve into old age was a definite plus.

The purported healthful influence of Tai Chi was the second factor that led me to the art. My readings promised that Tai Chi would promote muscle tone, relieved tensions due to stress, and aid in balance and good posture. These promises have not been false, and in fact, the first signs of improvement came within only a few months of beginning to learn the form. But it was the more esoteric promise of unimpeded chi flow enhancing my total well-being that really made me look closely at Tai Chi. What was this chi stuff? The books all said that every human, indeed all living things, are imbued with chi, but that, in the average person, it is undeveloped and undirected. Daily practice of Tai Chi and chi kung was said to enhance awareness of chi and give it conscious motivation. Though I had never heard of chi, it certainly sounded interesting.

And that brings me to the third factor that led me to take up Tai Chi. It's interesting. In the beginning you learn a somewhat complex series of movements that are a challenge to integrate into your present movement patterns. As you learn them, you begin to observe how they help you move better in daily life. At last you know how to perform the entire set of movements solo. You can feel the healthful benefits, you become more grounded in your movements, and you start to think, "Hey, I'm really getting this stuff." Then all of a sudden, you realize just how little you do know. To use a venerable Tai Chi simile, you're like a sculptor who has taken an unformed block of stone and roughed out the form within. But you've just taken the first step. From that point onward, you will constantly modify and improve the postures and stances, further hewing the stone into a recognizable and polished work of art.

And the beauty is that you work on yourself. You are the work of art. As you struggle with a particular posture or transition, you frequently struggle as much with psychological and emotional blockages as with physical ones. Release of those blockages and physical health go hand-in-hand in ways that are often as surprising as they are obvious once you've released them. For me, Tai Chi has only gotten more interesting, has only showed greater depth. If I've sometimes found daily practice tedious, it's usually because something greater is just around the corner. If I just walk a little farther though the postures, I'll round that corner.

The longer I do Tai Chi, the more I understand the term "Tai Chi player," for it does become joyous play. There are so many secrets embodied in the art that even after more than four decades of practicing and studying Tai Chi, I feel like I've only barely scratched the surface. Today, I find it more fascinating than ever.

Longevity and Tai Chi

Among the many benefits ascribed to Tai Chi Chuan is that of longevity. It is said that the art not only imparts health and well-being, it also contributes to a longer life in the practitioner. This idea, however, like the belief that anyone can learn and practice Tai Chi, is more myth than reality. If it were true that Tai Chi imparts a longer life, one might expect to see significantly increased life spans among the most celebrated masters of Tai Chi. This, however, does not bear out.

In his book *Tai Chi Dynamics: Principles of Natural Movement, Health, and Self-Development*, Robert Chuckrow lists the lifespans of thirty-two major Chinese Tai Chi masters who lived beween 1771 and 1997. Included among them are Yang Lu-chan, Yang Cheng-fu, Yang Pan-hou, Li I-yu, Sun Lu-tang, Cheng Man-ching, and T. T. Liang. This is how their ages at death break down: 50s: 8, 60s: 6, 70s: 10, 80s: 4, 90s: 2, 100s: 2. Yang Cheng-fu died at age 53 and Yang Pan-hou at age 55 (though I have heard that was suicide). Few people would have messed with these men during their prime, but their Tai Chi not only could not defeat death, it seemed to do little to stave it off.

Obviously, lifestyle has a lot to do with health. Yang Cheng-fu grew quite corpulent, and it is rumored that Cheng Man-ching was alcoholic. Others of these master might have smoked, drank, or eaten too much. It is true, though that the ages of the masters listed tend to increase toward the end of the list, which might be due to advances in medicine. On average, people who lived a century or more ago simply did not live as long as we do today. But except for the two who lived to be more than 100, the life spans of even the later practitioners are not any different than the current norms for non-practitioners. What, then should we make of the idea that Tai Chi imparts longevity?

Perhaps we should not think of longevity in terms of years lived but rather in terms of youthfulness. The truth is that Tai Chi will not appreciably increase the length of one's life any more than most exercise systems might. But it does something that most don't. It emphasizes the flexibility of the sinews—ligaments, tendons, and fascia. As people age, they not only lose muscle mass and tone, but their sinews tend to tighten, harden, and become stiff and brittle. But because Tai Chi trains the practitioner to move his or her body by using the sinews rather than muscles, these physiological structures are constantly being stretched and compressed, twisted and untwisted, keeping them flexible even into older age.

Thus, while Tai Chi might not impart a longer life, it assists one in maintaining the flexibility, pliability, and strength of the sinews. This imparts in the practitioner looser movements usually associated with youth. Hence, Tai Chi people seem to be younger than their calendar ages simply because they move like younger folks.

2. Chang San-feng: His Life and Deeds

An Apocryphal Biography of the Legendary Founder of Tai Chi Chuan

Compiled by Jack McGann and Christopher Dow

Chang San-feng is revered by practitioners of Tai Chi Chuan as the founder of the art. Maybe he actually lived, maybe he didn't. Maybe he created Tai Chi, then perhaps.... It doesn't really matter. His life and exploits form part of what the Chinese call "wild history." He is the Paul Bunyan of Tai Chi. Whatever the truth about his life, we know for certain that the person who first brought Tai Chi to the earthly plane couldn't have been merely a common man.

His Life

Chang San-feng was born sometime between 600 and 1600 AD, perhaps sometime during the Sung Dynasty, or maybe the Yuan Dynasty, but exactly at midnight on the fourth of April, 1247, and he lived precisely between the years 960 and 1126. His family came from I-Chou in the Liao-tung Peninsula.

He spent many years at the Temple of the Jade Void, becoming expert in Shaolin kung fu. Early on, it was discovered that he could recite Taoist classics after only a single reading. As he traveled, he became wise in the meditative and martial arts.

At the age of sixty-seven, he retired to the Wu Tang Mountains, where he built himself a cottage. At rest, he meditated, returning to the Original Source;

通微顯化張真人像

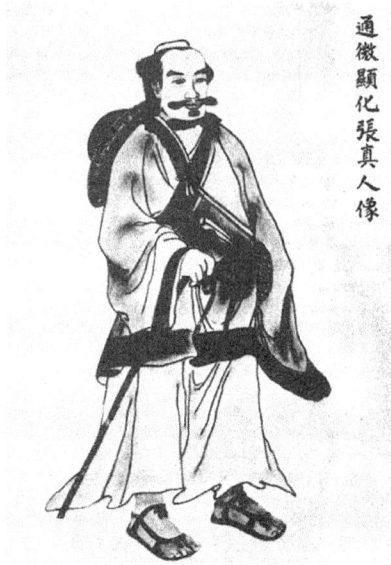

Figure 1.3 The supposed image of Chang San-feng, left, is probably not an accurate depiction. Chang, who was nicknamed Lar-tar (Sloppy) and La T'a (Dirty Fellow), was reputedly not nearly so neat and clean and was probably closer in appearance and dress to the image on the right.

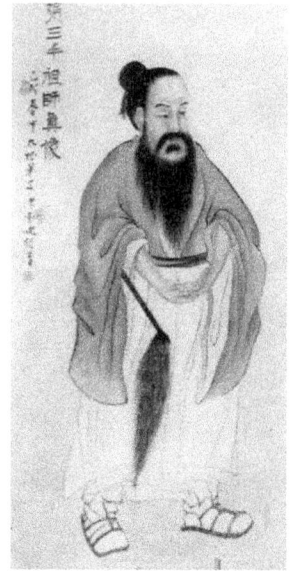

when active, he roamed the Three Mountains and the Five Peaks, gleaning the finest elements and subtle chi of Heaven and Earth and circulating them with breathing exercises. During this time, his reputation spread far and wide. The first Ming emperor sent a messenger to find him and bring him to court, but the errand was unsuccessful.

His Character and Appearance

Throughout his life, Chang took pains to conceal his achievements. He did not want to appear at court and so worked hard to seem mad. Everyone agrees that he did not keep himself neat and clean; Chang Lar-tar (Sloppy Chang) or La T'a (Dirty Fellow) often acted as if no one was around, spitting, farting, and scratching. He liked to tease people. He was very virtuous and often displayed such great mirth that is was impossible to remain melancholy in his presence. Winter and summer, he wore the same rude bamboo hat, the same old, ragged priest's robe. Instead of a staff, he carried a horsehair broom. Sometimes he would eat a bushel of food at a time, then again, he wouldn't eat for weeks. He never ate grains or cereals at all.

His picture can be seen at the White Cloud Temple in Beijing. He was seven feet tall, had bones like a crane; his posture was like a pine tree, his face round like an ancient moon, with kind brows and generous eyes and whiskers shaped like a spear; he was a big man, shaped like a turtle (a symbol of longevity), with a crane's back, large ears, round eyes, and beard like the tassel on a spear. He was very tall, his beard reached his navel, his hair touched the ground.

He had six hobbies: sword playing in moonlight, playing Tai Chi in the dark, mountain climbing on windy nights, reading the classics on rainy nights, meditating at midnight in the full moon, and playing the lute.

His Accomplishments

During his meditations in the Wu Tang Mountains, Chang was inspired to develop Tai Chi Chuan. One day, while reciting the classics, he heard a crane sing joyfully, like the sound of the zither. The Immortal came out of his hut to observe, and he saw the magpie peer at a snake on the ground. The snake darted hither and thither, coiling and recoiling. The raven attacked, and though the eagle struck over and over, it was unable to make a decisive strike.

After the several-hour encounter, the combatants disappeared. Like lightning, it struck Chang: The snake's coil was like the curve of the yin–yang and demonstrated the principle of the soft overcoming the hard, just as water eventually wears out rock, the tongue outlives the teeth, and the willow bends in the storm while the oak falls. From these insights, he developed the art of Tai Chi Chuan.

One day, the Immortal suddenly saw a burst of golden light where the mists shrouded the peaks. A thousand rays of chi spun and danced in the Great Void. He searched where the golden light touched down and found a mountain stream issuing from a cave. Approaching the cave, he saw two golden snakes with flashing eyes. He swished his horsehair duster and realized that they were really two spears of such quality that swords could not harm them. Master Chang also discovered in the cave a glowing book of songs and poems from which he extracted the essence, transforming them into the postures of the art of Tai Chi spear.

His Exploits

Chang used the movement Diagonal Flying to break firewood in the forest, and he had a large pet ape who collected the firewood for him. In fact, the ape so often had an opportunity to watch the Master practice that, in faithful imitation, it developed a simian version of Tai Chi.

Upon being attacked by a python, Chang grasped the serpent at either end, and using the technique of Parting the Wild Horse's Mane, he tore it into pieces. Once, encountering a tiger in the mountains, he applied the skill of Bend the Bow to Shoot the Tiger—first he turned to avoid the tiger's rush, then grasping the two hind legs as the beast passed, he tore it in half.

He could travel two hundred miles in one day. He was so light-footed that he left no footprints in the snow, but his internal energy was so strong that paths would appear in the snow, melted from the heat he generated. His robes rustled as he meditated, and the walls shook. Carrying his horsehair duster, he could out-walk everyone, going a thousand miles at a time. They say he lived for two hundred years and possessed such powerful energy that the sick would collect dirt from his body, roll it into balls, and eat it to cure disease.

His words have come down to us as the "Tai Chi Ching," always the first-quoted in every collection of the Tai Chi Classics.

His Further Exploits

Once, when members of the royal Mongolian family of the Yuan Dynasty were hunting in the mountains, they ran across Chang as he was picking herbs. Though aware that the Mongolians were excellent bowmen, he was offended by their pomposity, so that when they ordered him to leave, he refused. Angrily he said to the prince, "Your highness hunts with a bow and arrow, but I use only bare hands." Suddenly two hawks flew by, and Chang leapt up, caught them, then dropped silently to the ground. Chang stood a bird in each of his palms, but no matter how hard they tried to fly away, they could not escape, such was his yielding ability. Then Chang said to the shocked prince, "I have mercy on living creatures and do not want to hurt the birds." He let the birds fly away. One of the guards was so incensed that he drew his bow and shot an arrow at Chang, but the Master caught the arrow in his teeth. Then, holding the arrow in his fingers, he threw it at a tree, where it buried deep into the wood. "I have no need of violent weapons," he commented dryly.

Some time after creating Tai Chi, Chang was ordered to appear at the court of the Emperor Tai-tsu. On the way, while crossing a bridge, he was attacked by a band of one hundred brigands who thought him easy prey. Within moments, the fight was over, all the outlaws lying unconscious on the ground. Chang walked away unscathed. Later, when the outlaws awoke, they swore that the old man hadn't even used his arms or legs but had merely shrugged them aside as they attacked, flinging them into unconsciousness. When Chang reached the palace, the emperor conferred on him the title, "T'ung-wei'hsien'hua chen-jen," which meant, "The spiritual man who understands the power of the occult."

No one is certain when Chang died, or even if he did. Robert W. Smith, writing as John F. Gilbey, tells in his book, *The Way of the Warrior*, of learning about a man named Lu, living in New York City during the 1950s and 1960s, whose life so imitated Chang San-feng that he might have been the Master himself.[1]

Part II

Miscellaneous Matters

3. The Paradox of Violence

Where does the truth of martial arts lie: in the practice room or on the street? Is it in the perseverance and dedication to form or in gut-level spontaneous violence and backlash? This is a seemingly eternal topic of debate whose very importance is demonstrated by its imperishability. Yet, can there be a correct answer to an incorrect question? A recent incident brought to my attention—and dismay—some of the paradoxes involved in this issue.

I was on the patio, practicing my Tai Chi form, when two boys, ten or so years old, approached the fence and started watching me.

"You doing karate?" the bigger one asked.

"No, a kind of kung fu," I replied, continuing with my form.

"Is it like karate?" the smaller one wanted to know.

"Karate is Japanese, kung fu is Chinese."

Pause.

"You do it every day?" The smaller one again.

"Yes."

Pause.

"Do you use it for self-defense?" asked the bigger one.

"Well, I guess I could if I had to."

"I got something for self-defense, too," the bigger one said.

I stopped moving as I saw him tentatively reach into his pocket, a sinking feeling in my gut. I wasn't frightened, for his movement wasn't threatening, just wrenched to my roots, knowing he was going to proudly show me something I didn't really want to see.

Almost shyly he dragged the butterfly knife out of his pocket and awkwardly displayed it. It flopped loosely as he held the hinge pinched between his forefinger and thumb. He hadn't even had it locked closed in his pocket, though he'd probably become all-too-expert with it all too soon. The late afternoon sun gleamed on the swinging handles, the dangling blade. He smiled.

Even the best of us have a hard time being brilliant on the spur of the moment. Besides, how do you explain to a ten-year-old stranger from another world that he's got it all wrong? All I could do was look him in the eye and say in a sad tone, "That's great if you always have it, if you always want to hurt someone."

His shy, proud smile faded as his forehead creased in a puzzled expression.

I looked at that boy, taking in the terrible dichotomy of the innocence of the child, the violence of the blade. How easily they could assume each other's roles. How easily human violence can wield innocent matter to destructive ends. How easily the knife invites—perhaps invokes—that violence.

Suddenly he was nudged in the ribs by the smaller kid, who jerked his head. "Let's go."

And off they ran, the bigger kid stuffing the deadly butterfly back into his pocket. I stepped forward, wanting to yell, "Come back. Let me tell you about self-control, about real self-defense!" But they had disappeared into the dusk.

Troubled, I returned to my practice, thinking that the truth of fighting and violence lies not in locations and situations but in the more intangible latitudes and inaccessible occurrences of the hearts, minds, and souls of human beings.

> The sage is he who has attained the central point of the Wheel and remains bound to the "Unvarying Mean," in indissoluble union with the Origin, partaking of its immutability and imitating its non-acting activity. He who has reached the highest degree of emptiness, will be secure in repose. To return to the root is to enter into the state of repose, that is, to throw off the bonds of things transitory and contingent.
>
> —Taoist Sage
> in J.E. Cirlot,
> *A Dictionary of Symbols*

4. Christianity versus Chi

I once wrote a review of *Chinese Wand Exercises*, by Bruce L. Johnson, whose history was quite remarkable. But one element of it gave me pause. Johnson learned judo and other martial arts in Japan and China right after World War II and, on his return to the United States, became friends with Bruce Lee and other members of the then relatively small U.S. kung fu community. But later in life, Johnson became a born-again Christian and promptly rejected his martial arts past.

"These things are not from God," he once said, referring to chi energy and the martial arts. "God is not in the business of mystical energies or the occult. I no longer practice the martial arts.... As a Christian, I cannot in good conscience, teach or recommend the martial arts to others."[1] Johnson's conversion under this mindset was a blow to the martial arts, for Johnson, the final grandmaster of Chinese wand exercises, took a great number of these exercises to the grave.

I've heard this sort of thing before from some Christians: The Eastern martial arts, chi kung, yoga, and meditation—and the energies they foster—are anti-Christian and even demonic. After reading Johnson's statements, I decided to do a little research into the matter. A cursory look online confirmed that a great number of Christians do believe that these energies are corrupting at best and Satanic at worst.

These ideas were perfectly typified in 2010, when Reverend David Rhodes of the All Saints Church Hall in Totley, Yorkshire, England, forbade the church hall from being used for Tai Chi classes. The practice was, he said, anti-Christian.[2] Rhodes' rejection, bland though it is, is merely the tip of a more treacherous iceberg. So, before I begin my evaluation, let me expose more of the mass of this frozen belief by presenting the opinions of some Christians regarding these matters in their own words.

By definition alone, the idea of chi is not compatible with the Christian faith," one website states. "A foundational doctrine of Christianity is that God created all things through Jesus (see Genesis 1:1 and John 1:1-4). It is God who gives life, and by God, through Jesus, all things are sustained (see Psalm 147:9 and Colossians 1:16-17).... Some may argue that chi is just a different term for the 'life' that God breathed into Adam (Genesis 2:7). But we can't transplant the term chi into the Christian faith because the philosophy behind chi (Taoism) is also incompatible with Christianity. For example, the Taoist view of 'God' is that each person has his or her own definition of what 'god' is, and each definition is perfectly acceptable—neither right nor wrong. In the Christian faith, God is not defined by people's perceptions. Rather, He reveals who He is to us (see Jeremiah 29:13-14). While God is infinite and beyond human understanding, He has revealed certain things about Himself and is able to be known personally. In Christianity, Jesus Christ is the only way to a real relationship with God (see John 14:5-7).[3]

The website of the Christian Research Institute presents three views on the practice of martial arts by Christians:

1. "Because of its unchristian origin (Eastern mysticism), no martial art form should be practiced by Christians."
2. "As long as the Christian divorces the religious aspects (Eastern mysticism) from the martial arts, he or she may practice them." The site then goes on to list a number of martial arts and ranks them according to how easily one can "divorce the religious aspects" from them. Judo/Jujutsu, karate, and Taekwondo, all having a primarily physical rather than spiritual component, make the cautious cut, but Aikido, kung fu, Ninjitsu, and Tai Chi are all too steeped in Eastern mysticism to be "safe" for Christian consumption.
3. "The martial arts are not compatible with Christianity because of their violent nature." The author goes on to say that while self-defense is generally acceptable, Christians probably ought to turn the other cheek instead.[4]

The author then writes, "The Christian must realize that because this is a controversial area, he or she must be careful not to cause a weaker Christian to stumble by practicing a martial art (Rom. 14). Second, (primarily for youths), the Christian must guard against the temptation of starting fights. Third, the Christian should not allow a martial art to overshadow or detract from his Christian commitments."

The Women of Grace organization has this to say in a blog titled, *Why Tai Chi and Catholicism Don't Mix*:

> Tai chi is based on the existence of a life force energy that science has never been able to substantiate…. The belief that a life force energy pervades all of nature is known as pantheism and is not compatible with Christianity. The Pontifical Councils for Culture and Irreligious Dialogue called this impersonal energy force a "New Age god," in their document, *Jesus Christ the Bearer of the Water of Life*…. 'This is very different from the Christian understanding of God as the maker of heaven and earth and the source of all personal life.[5]

The ironically named *The Free Press* website has an article titled "Tai chi: occult, dangerous and not for Christians—we answer our critics," that reads:

> [God] does NOT approve it! It is based on a pagan belief that "chi" is a universal force. This is not true. There is no "chi," but the real force that holds the universe together is the will of the Lord Jesus Christ, who made everything and holds all things together (Colossians 1:17). So right there at the very foundations of tai chi, you have a lie.[6]

The text goes on to state: "The slow motion exercises of tai chi supposedly open pathways for the 'chi' energy to flow. This should set alarm bells ringing if you are a Christian! Why would you want to control some supernatural power and make it flow through your own body? This is absolutely not of God! If you do open a spiritual pathway, something might just come in!" It should be noted that The Free Press website also has this headline on its front page: "Proof positive—the Catholic Church is not Christian! It is a counterfeit."

Yoga and meditation fare no better than Tai Chi or other martial arts, with the detractors using much the same arguments. And occasionally, the detractors are even harsher regarding Kundalini energy, which often is described as serpentine. Considering how much Christians hate and fear the serpent, it's no surprise that some consider Kundalini to be particularly Satanic and leading to demonic possession.[7,8,9,10]

If you think you had a hard time reading these statements without your hackles rising, just remember: I had to type up this stuff. And I read even more. But now that the principle Christian arguments against esoteric energies and the practices that foster them are on the table, let me begin dismantling them.

1. Esoteric energies are not compatible with the Christian faith, the first quote above says, because God created all things through Jesus.

The writer cites Genesis 1:1 and John 1:1-4 to substantiate this statement, but unfortunately, neither passage mentions Jesus. They say that God is the one who did all the creating. Jesus doesn't even make an appearance until the New Testament, which begins, according to Christian history, about six thousand years after the God's six days of labor and one of rest. This makes these passages useless as authoritative sources for this argument, even if one were inclined to take the Bible as literal history. So, I want to know if God personally told the writer that he doesn't like chi energy, or if the writer is just assuming so, since the writer's sources don't back him up. And to claim that God only makes his will known through Jesus Christ is also to say that the Old Testament is not a reliable back-up for any argument since everything that transpires in it occurs prior to Christ's birth, and he isn't even mentioned much in it. In addition, if all things (reality) were created by God, then he created chi as much as he did the heavens and the earth or plants and animals.

2. Chi is not the same as the God's "breath of life."

Well, first of all, was the writer present when God did that breathing? If not, then the writer does not really know the exact nature of that breath of life—or even what the term actually means—any more than he understands the nature of chi. But presumably, the writer means that God inspired the life of living creatures by investing in each of them a small measure of spirit. It seems to me that only an obtuse or exclusivist individual would argue that the breath of life imparted by the Tao is fundamentally different from the breath of life imparted by God. Both are synonymous with the life force imparted into mortal creatures by the unnamable, unknowable universal force behind, beneath, around, and through all of reality.

3. Some individuals insist that chi cannot be the same as God's breath because Taoist philosophy has an unchristian origin and is not compatible
   with Christianity.

Right off the bat, this does not logically follow. Christians readily take advantage
of modern science, technology, and medicine, none of which have a Christian
origin and all of which are based on tenets that are largely incompatible with
Christian beliefs. Further, though Christians might deny it, there can be more
than one road to the same destination. In any case, Christianity, itself, has its
roots in Judaism, which isn't exactly Christian, either. And add the fact that Jesus disappeared into the desert—and very possibly traveled to the East, where
he picked up some of those unchristian ideas that thoroughly informed his belief system—and it seems that the first part of the writer's argument fails since
even Christianity itself is, at least partly, of unchristian origins.

   Besides, there are a number of compelling parallels between the basic tenets
of Christianity and Taoism. God is the supreme force, creator, and intelligence
behind the universe, and he is unknowable. Likewise, the Tao is the supreme
force, creator, and intelligence behind the universe and also is unknowable. And
both God and the Tao accord humans free will to follow a path back to the creator force or to deviate from that path.

   The principle difference is that Christians believe in a personal God who
watches over—and judges—every individual, while the Tao is much more impersonal and might not pay particular attention to any one person. And for the
Tao, there is no judgement because the Tao simply *is* and is beyond judgement.
But I have to say that, even if the Christian God does watch over us all individ-
ually, he rarely steps in to right wrongs, avert disaster, or relieve suffering. In
fact, since all this stuff goes on all the time despite multitudes of prayers for
relief, God seems just as remote as the Tao and not at all engaged with people
on a personal level. But I suppose the Christian could assert that he feels the
spirit of God within his breast. Guess what? Me, too, only I call it the Tao. And
please don't tell me that my personal sense of God is somehow bogus or inferi-
or to yours, or I might level the same accusation at you.

   For the Christian, God, in the first moment of creation, separated the cosmos into pairs of fundamental polar opposites: the light and darkness and the
heavens and the earth. Kind of seems to be the same thing as: The Tao moved,
creating the yin and yang. From there, Adam (yang) and Eve (yin) populated the
world, just as, in Taoism, the interplay of yang and yin created the many and
diverse forms of reality. Even disregarding the findings of genetic studies of
the human race, certainly Adam and Eve can't have been actual humans who
physically procreated to produce the human race. I know that the arguments

below are old, but if they need to be raised again to beat back old but persistent canards, so be it.

If Adam and Eve were the first people, and they produced only two sons, one of whom murdered the other, then that's pretty much the end since Cain didn't have a woman companion, and it takes two to raise little Cains. But, oh yeah, some Christians say that there were other people who helped generate more people, but if so, exactly where did those other people come from? If they were not Adam and Eve's children but were created by God after he put the first couple on the earth, then they—and we—aren't direct descendants of Adam and Eve and so should not have inherited their original sin. Assuming you inherit such things like you do your genetic makeup or cultural proclivities.

But the genesis of these other people isn't in Genesis, and if the Bible is the final and ultimate authority, then all we have is Cain to begin the population explosion that's now eating humanity alive. You can see the problem there. But let's say that Adam and Eve did have other children who then populated the earth. That means that we are all, every one of us, the product of incest. It's even a sort of parthenogenetic incest since Eve came straight from Adam's rib. If humankind is cursed with original sin, it's no wonder: We're all inbred hillbillies. But if we're all formed from Adam's exact DNA, how come we don't all look like Adam and each other? And what about Eve? Did she look just like Adam since she was his clone? Or was that rib…different, somehow? Must have been.

Taoism does not adhere to the doctrine of original sin. It just assumes that people are simply unadvanced and are bound to make mistakes. Thus it does not offer forgiveness or salvation—or even damnation—merely another chance to do better. But there are further parallels between it and Christianity. Christ's principles of peace and good will toward others, non-violence, and finding a true path to oneness with the creator are not fundamentally different from the tenets of Taoism. But Christian critics of chi energy use a mischaracterization of Taoism to bolster their argument. This mischaracterization is exhibited in the first passage above: "The Taoist view of 'God' is that each person has his or her own definition of what 'god' is, and each definition is perfectly acceptable—neither right nor wrong."

This is, at root, false. In the first place, Taoism doesn't encourage you to make up a concept of God or deity from whole cloth. Instead, it suggests a method—or Way—to conduct one's life in order to achieve oneness with the whole of creation—at the head of which, of course, must be God—or the Tao. Each person, being an individual, finds that Way on their own and in their own way. I fail to see how this could be otherwise since humanity is clearly not just clones of Adam with identical DNA, nor are we possessed of an overt group mind, like some insects, that dictates specifics of internalized belief, behavior, and revelation. Each of us are different and must find what we seek—be it God or some lesser goal—on our own and through our own comprehension and our own means and methods. I'm reminded here of the saying: Do what you can with what you've got.

And despite writing, "In the Christian faith, God is not defined by people's perceptions," the writer goes on to say, "Rather, He reveals who He is to us. While God is infinite and beyond human understanding, He has revealed certain things about Himself and is able to be known personally." Isn't that pretty much the same as finding your own personal understanding of or connection to God? If God is going to reveal himself to me—at least in small-enough measure that my dinky human psyche can withstand that revelation—how can I experience it other than with my perceptions, colored by my background, life experiences, intelligence and education, and so forth? Revelation, like reality, can only be taken in via perception, otherwise it is a wind that we do not feel within the walls of our house.

And of course revelation must be personal because it is a person who experiences it via their perceptions. And each person, being an individual, comes to an individual comprehension of revelation—his or her own definition of God. And seriously, is God going to falsify my perceptions of him? If there's any falsification, it'll come from my own weaknesses, foibles, ignorance, stubbornness, and so forth, all of which filter my understanding of God and his revelations into a personal understanding of deity.

I'd bet that if you asked ten Christians their exact definition of God, there would be some variance. Aren't those variances manifestations of a revelation of God from a personal perspective? In other words, each of us—Christian, Taoist, or whatever—has a personal definition of what God is. And all those definitions bear equal weight since it is the fate of humankind not to know its origins or its fate—and, in any case, each and every one of our personal definitions are wrong, if for no other reason than that they are inadequate in every way. Apparently the writer would not agree since he thinks he's clenched it when he finishes: "In Christianity, Jesus Christ is the only way to a real relationship with God." Maybe, but I kind of doubt it. Was Christ saying that you have to worship him as a deity in order to be saved, or was he saying that he knew the way—the means and methods—to salvation (oneness with deity) and that he was willing to show others how to travel that same path?

Call me a Gnostic (though I prefer Taoist), but from my experience, one can have a direct connection to the greater spiritual reality—call it God, the Tao, Allah, or whatever you want. But then, Christian churches have always been about hierarchy, permission, and limited access to deity. It's a pay-to-play scheme that threatens eternal perdition for failure to adhere to religion's all-too-human restrictions, no matter how good you are otherwise. After all, if everyone can have direct access to God—the Tao—who needs preachers or churches? Besides, I'm not quite so willing to damn the 99.999 percent of all the people who've ever lived who weren't Christians and let Christians off the hook when they don't seem to be superior in any way, including holiness, to anyone else.

4. A Christian may practice the martial arts if he or she eschews the esoteric energies.

Well, gosh: Let's play *Monopoly* without money or build a brick wall without mortar. Half the point of practicing the martial arts is to develop chi energy! Maybe more than half, in the long run. Anything else is just moving muscle without higher dimensions. Not that exercise isn't good, but exercise with higher dimensions is better. And when you get old, muscles may wither, but strong chi can help you remain more healthy and vital.

5. The martial arts have a violent nature that conflicts with the Christian tenet of turning the other cheek.

I can't really argue with the first part of this statement. The martial arts are definitely violent, or can be. They are, after all, arts of Mars, the god of war. But it also is possible to practice them for health, increased internal energy, self-development, and spiritual development rather than for fighting. And certainly, chi kung, yoga, and meditation are inherently peaceful and non-violent and do not have a combat motive or methodology though they all also strongly develop chi energy.

The hypocrisy of this criticism of chi is stunning. For more than a millennium—and often on massive scales—Christians have actively engaged in intentional violence, hatred, murder, genocide, torture, pogroms, and the destruction of historical and cultural artifacts. Just a cursory glance at the Christian Right in America and its political and cultural agendas shows its members to be callous, violence prone, exclusionary, and heavily armed. So much for turning the other cheek. Besides, Christians have fought in every war available to them, and they've even fomented quite a few of their own, including several hundred years of Crusades that largely sparked the anti-Western sentiment and conflict in the Middle East that continues today. Why do they fight? "Well, it's my Christian duty."

6. Practicing martial arts can tempt other Christian believers to stumble into negative behavior.

In my experience, those who stumble into negative behavior, at least for any extended period of time, probably want to stumble in that direction. And pretending to be good doesn't make you so, particularly if your actions speak otherwise.

Along with this criticism is another: that martial arts abilities and the commitment necessary to develop them, can cause the practitioner to be distracted from one's commitment to the feeling of oneness with God. I guess that slavish adherence to Sunday afternoon football, which is little more than stylized warfare, also might qualify as a distraction, too, especially on the Sabbath. In any case, if a given practice can impart health, make you feel good inside and out, and lend a sense of oneness with creation and with your fellow humans, why would you automatically assume that God did not intend for you to undertake that practice or believe that, somehow, it must be evil?

7. Chi is not real, but a fantasy that has not been substantiated by science. The real force that binds the universe is not chi but the will of Jesus Christ.

Wow, is this an amusing argument, or what? Christians tend to denigrate science at every turn when it posits an Earth that existed for billions of years before humans came on the scene, Darwinism, or many other scientific principles that conflict with Biblical literalism. Many Christians believe that humans and dinosaurs walked the earth together, for example, willfully ignoring the blatant evidence that lies there for all to see. Furthermore, science can't substantiate either the existence of God or the will of Jesus Christ that Christians say is what is holding the universe together.

Any good scientist will tell you there are many things and forces in the universe that have not yet been examined—or even perceived—by science, much less explained. And while it's probably true that not everything can be explained by scientists or anyone else, good scientists also will admit that it's impossible to prove a negative—that is, you can't prove that something isn't or can't be. You only can prove what is, and even that's pretty hard to do, especially when a large contingent of the population won't consider any scientific evidence much less accept it. And actually, some scientists *are* actively working toward an understanding of chi as a natural force produced by the body and have made considerable headway. (More on that below.)

And finally, if the will of Jesus Christ is what holds the universe together, I guess we don't need the strong nuclear force or gravity, the former of which binds atomic structure and the latter of which binds the macro structure of the universe. I suppose the Christian might argue that gravity and the strong nuclear force—two of the four fundamental forces of the universe—are simply the manifestations of that will of Christ that's holding the universe together. But if so, then why isn't chi also a legitimate a force, especially if it is, essentially, electromagnetism, which is another of the four fundamental universal forces? (See below for more on the idea that chi is electromagnetism.)

8. A belief in chi is equivalent to a belief in pantheism.

This criticism stems from the Christian idea that every other religion the world has ever seen anywhere is pagan, corrupt, delusional, and dangerous. The idea of pantheism is, it seems, a total anathema to the Christian, who worships a single, all-powerful deity and denies that other single, all-powerful deities also exist—or perhaps, that all such deities are, in fact, the same deity in different guises.

But does the Christian God really exist as a singular deity? What about the Trinity of three separate though interconnected aspects of deity? What about all those angels and seraphim, those devils and demons? Aren't those basically elements of deity (yang) and anti-deity (yin) working their wiles upon humanity no less than the pantheons of Greek, Roman, Hindu, and other religions? No religion asks that its supreme deity do all the work all by itself, not even Christianity. Besides, do you think that it's actually possible for measly little humans to comprehend even the slightest portion of deity or what it wants? For the most part, we can't even comprehend ourselves beyond our own dimly-envisioned wants, much less someone else so much more grand.

But by pantheism, the Christian also means the belief that all of nature is imbued with living vitality, from the highest creature to the lowest. Most pantheists include plants, and some even inanimate objects. Of course, Christians also deny that any creatures but man have souls, and they wouldn't even consider that inanimate object could house some sort of vitality or energy. This is at odds, however, with a great number of other religions and spiritual systems that, each in its own way, acknowledges esoteric energies and believes that all of manifest reality is imbued with this spectrum of spiritual energy. This energy, they say, is the way—the means and methods—creation uses to manifest.

Even science accepts the idea that the universe is imbued with vitality—or energy—though science would tend to dispute with religion as to this vitality's nature, origins, development, and meaning. For science, this inspiriting vitality is the natural system of organization that creates a given set of sub-atomic "particles" out of vibrations, then arranges these several vibrations into various larger groups of interacting vibrations that form atomic structures. Those structures are the elements, the basic manifestations of reality. From there on, the structure of the universe is more a matter of mechanics—adding, subtracting, and combining—to create the more sophisticated aspects of reality, with human intervention overlaying natural constructs with the tools and machinery of our civilizations. For religion, the cause is…. Well, plug in your own name for it; I like the Tao, which split into the yin and yang, whose mutual interplay creates multifold reality. Besides, science already has proven that energy does pervade the universe. Even a vacuum contains a steady state of energetic activity.

Isn't it interesting that, in a sense, science validates Taoism? According to science, reality is the product of vibration, which is, in and of itself, a yin/yang state. The only real questions are: What is the substance that is vibrating, who or what set the vibrations going, and how and why was that done? Probably we'll never know the answers to the last three of those questions, but science might yet identify the underlying substance with which the Tao's alternating yin-yang pulsations interact. And though science has not yet specifically identified chi energy to the satisfaction of all (or most), it does parallel Taoist philosophy regarding the origin and sub-structure of reality.

9. Why would anyone want to open themselves to chi energy, which is tantamount to a supernatural power, and allow it to flow inside them?

I fully admit that chi is a supernatural force. How could I not? It, like all of reality, is a mystery for which we have no definitive cause and only the barest understanding. I could say with some accuracy that the whole of reality itself is nothing but an overwhelming supernatural force. And the same with God.

But the Pontifical Council for Culture and Irreligious Dialogue says that chi is an impersonal energy and a "New Age god." What, then, about the strong nuclear force, the weak nuclear force, gravity, and electromagnetism? These are the four fundamental forces of nature that are recognized by science as being irreducible (as far as we currently know) to any more basic force. All act in a way that is invisible and unknown to normal perceptions. But two of them—gravity and electromagnetism—can be sensed by the human body, and the other two can be detected by scientific instruments. Are these invisible, imperceptible, and impersonal energies also false "New Age gods?" And what if chi is really electromagnetism? Would it still be considered a false god, or would it be considered a natural force that, though impersonal, remains fundamental?

There is, in fact, strong evidence that points to chi being electromagnetic in nature. See my book, *The Wellspring: An Inquiry into the Nature of Chi*, for a more comprehensive explanation of what chi is, how it is generated, and how it can be better channeled through the body, but in short, chi likely consists of the electromagnetic fields that surround our nerves and is powered by the movement of nerve impulses.

These electromagnetic fields constantly circulate through the torso, flowing along with the bioelectrical impulses that are generated in the intestines by the physiological action of breathing and are then pushed up the spine and through the brain. Along the spine are two major nerve "intersections." At the sacral plexus, located in the lower back, some of the bioelectric nerve impulses and attendant electromagnetic fields are pushed into the legs, and at the brachial plexus, located between the shoulders, a similar things happens for the arms.

In the limbs, these fields are quiescent when the body is still, and they move when the nervous system impels movement and sends impulses down the nerves. Chi is not some alien force that one creates or inserts or invites into oneself. Instead, it is part of and engendered by our living bodies. It is simply a pulse of electromagnetic energy that follows nerve impulses. If you do not have chi running through your body, that means you no longer have bioelectrical impulses running through your nerves. In that case, yep: You're dead.

10. If you open a spiritual pathway, you might be invaded by an evil force.

If you don't open a spiritual pathway, you will never be invaded by good forces, either, or reach oneness with the universal spirit, whatever you name it. The simple fact is that humans are intended and largely engineered to engage in spiritual advancement—to work our way toward God, so to speak—and developing a higher spiritual consciousness and abilities are inevitable as we grow spiritually. Yes, perhaps evil forces can attempt to invade a person who is working to become a better or greater person. (See the essay, "Haunted: No. 10," in my *Book of Curiosities: Adventures in the Paranormal.*) At all levels of life, from the mundane to the spiritual, one is subjected to pernicious or evil influences, but that doesn't mean they must be allowed admittance or control. If evil forces can invade a person, most likely it's a person who is willing to be invaded rather than one who is not.

Humanity exhibits a range of powers, abilities, and proclivities, all of which can be developed and enhanced. The simple fact is that the real issue surrounding chi energy isn't the energy itself but the ways in which it is wielded by those who develop it. Developing spiritual energies and opening yourself to spiritual forces is no different than developing other parts of your being. To say that a person who develops his or her chi will automatically misuse this power or invite demonic spirits is like saying that a body builder will always use the muscles he's strengthened to bully weaker people or that an intelligent person will inevitably use the knowledge he's gained to manipulate others.

A good strong man opts to use his strength to protect, and a good intelligent man uses his knowledge for the betterment of humankind. Here's the question: If someone gave you super powers, would you become a super hero or a super villain? Would you use your power to better others as well as yourself, or would you use it solely for your own ends and to subjugate others and exact revenge? Your answer will tell you if evil influences will prevail over your spirit, whether or not you develop chi energy.

The danger of misuse of chi power in olden China was dealt with by kung fu masters who tested the character of their students as much as they challenged their physical abilities. But even this practice couldn't prevent evil or corrupt people from learning and developing these powers for negative ends. Don't forget Shaolin's evil monk, Bai Mai! Such is life and the nature of reality. Some of us humans are good, some bad, and most are somewhere in between.

The truth is, it is hard enough to control one's own impulses and change oneself for the better, but it is impossible to do those things for others. All we can really do to change others is to be the change we want to see and to exhibit that better behavior in the hopes that others might emulate it. So, just because someone else uses a strength or power for negative purposes doesn't mean I have to do the same, even if I gain the ability to do so. When I get my chi flowing more powerfully and freely, it enables me to live life more robustly, and it also gives me something healthful and spiritually important to share with others.

One of the great ironies of Christian rejection of esoteric energy is that each and every human being has chi flowing in them at all times. For most people, this flow goes unnoticed and unheeded, but it is there, nonetheless. Chi-training exercises do not "introduce" some sort of weird, alien force into the body but simply encourage the practitioner to consciously sense, amplify, store, and manipulate an energy that is always present within the body and to open the body to this flow, which has healing properties. If you fear the idea of chi flowing inside you, you might as well fear the idea of blood flowing through your veins.

A second, and perhaps greater, irony is that Christian ministers and congregations regularly employ various methods to unconsciously unify and harness the diverse chi fields of worshippers during ceremonies. Let me begin explaining this through a bit of a detour:

In the summer of 1970, friends and I attended a music festival dubbed the Powder Ridge Rock Festival, which was held at the Powder Ridge Ski Area in Middlefield, Connecticut. This was a year after the Woodstock Music Festival, which I also attended, and my friends and I were hoping for something similar to occur at Powder Ridge, but that was not to be the case. The festival wasn't really a music festival at all, but a mob rip-off. The promoters rented the ski area during the off-season and sold many thousands of tickets but never booked any of the bands that they advertised would play. In the end, the desperate townspeople, anxious to avert a hippie riot (!), allowed in a couple of ice-cream trucks whose generators provided electricity to a makeshift stage where the folk singer, Melanie, and some local bands played to a massive crowd arrayed up the hill of the ski slope.

My friend and I did not sit in the crowd but occupied a sort of little nook in the tree line off to one side. The crowd spread out below, in front of, and above us, but we weren't actually part of it. During the time the technicians were wiring the trucks and hooking up the amplifiers, occasional bursts of static or the peal of a power chord from one of the guitars would blare out, and each time, a wave of energy would ripple through the crowd as it worked its way up the slope. These waves were tangible, feeling like a surge of excitement each time one passed, and we could see the people in the crowd react to this wave by becoming more physically animated as it crested over them, then less so as it passed on up the slope.

At the same time, someone had brought in a huge inflated ball and given it to the audience to play with. When I say huge, I mean really big—ten or more feet in diameter. It probably was one of those weather balloons advertised in the back pages of comic books and men's magazines. This ball wasn't fully filled with air, so its skin wasn't taut like a sport's ball but was somewhat slack. It kind of looked like the big ball that would chase #6 every time he tried to leave the Island in the '60s TV show, *The Prisoner*, and it had the same function here in pacifying the potentially unruly. This ball was being bounced into the air and passed around overhead by the audience, and as it moved over the crowd, I could feel ripples of excitement from the people underneath it radiate outward and propagate in whatever direction the ball took.

I realized that I was witnessing a more benign version of the collective madness that can grip a crowd and turn it into a riotous mob. I didn't know about chi at the time, but I recognized that some sort of hidden human energy—arcane but transmittable—was involved in these waves and ripples of excitement that collectively gripped the audience when the members were mutually focused in some specific way.

Memories of this event submerged as life went on, but after I'd been doing tai chi for about ten years, I was reminded of it in a way that gave me greater understanding of the phenomenon. At the time, I was involved in a video production company, and one of my jobs entailed videotaping a celebration at a fairly large charismatic church. The celebration began with half-a-dozen amateur-hour sorts of performances before moving on to a sermon and the singing of hymns.

During the amateur-hour performances, the atmosphere in the hall wasn't much different than for any other performance venue, but as soon as the sermon and the singing began, the atmosphere changed radically. It literally became charged with electricity as the entire congregation began swaying and moving to the rhythms of the preacher's voice and the hymns. "Do you feel it, brothers and sisters?" the preacher called out. "The spirit of God is with us!"

Well, yes, I felt it, but it wasn't the spirit of God, exactly. It was a manifestation of the unified chi fields of the entire audience moving in synchronization, producing a powerful physical, emotional, and psychic effect. I suppose you could categorize this unified energy as the spirit of God since chi is, at root, a manifestation of God's "breath of life," but I don't think it would be correct to draw that exact parallel. This same unified energy is also what powers destructive mobs.

You can even feel in when you're sitting in a movie theater and the entire audience is gripped with similar emotions. It's said that Helen Keller liked to go to the movies despite being blind and deaf. She could, she said, feel the emotions of the audience. It's a power that is unconsciously (at least for the most part) manipulated by individuals and groups who perform in front of any large crowd. "Okay, now!" yells the rock singer. "Put your hands together...!" Or the lead guitarist plays a power chord that sends a wave of energy right through everybody all at once, boosting the energy level in the auditorium. It's also the feeling you get when practicing Tai Chi in groups, and the unified movements of all the attendant chi fields synchronize into a gestalt that permeates the whole group. Christian churches generate this gestalt on a regular basis through focused group attention, kneeling and rising together in conjunction with prayer, unified chanting of prayers and singing of hymns emotionally bolstered by organ music, and sometimes swaying or dancing. The cadence adopted by many preachers also uses its rhythms—and call-and-response—to focus and collectively move a congregation.

I've spent a large amount of time on the question of chi as it relates to Christian beliefs, and some might think that Islam, being similar to Christianity in its roots, would have very similar attitudes. Interestingly, though, Islam has a somewhat less vitriolic response to these energies than does Christianity. But even so, fundamentalist Islamic writers on the subject frequently warn that the practice of martial arts, chi kung, meditation, and yoga can open one up to energies that one can't handle, leading to mental and psychic disturbances, or to outright possession by jinns—Islam's version of demons. Fear of the latter seems to be one of the greatest Islamic impediment to developing chi or Kundalini power.[11,12,13]

Perhaps it is true that chi and Kundalini—which likely are different manifestations of the same energy—and the practices that can strengthen them—martial arts, chi kung, yoga, and so forth—are anti-Christian. I don't mean by that that they are deliberately antagonistic to Christianity, but that their concepts are more inclusive of the actual nature of reality, which is less narrowly defined than it is in the Christian belief system. Most religions and spiritual systems that rely on the concept of chi (ki, prana, etc.) say it is a powerful energy in the body that is part of the natural spectrum of being: The soul inspires the spirit, the spirit informs the mind, the mind motivates the chi, and the chi moves the body.

Practices and exercises for chi development state that chi can be enhanced, circulated within the body, and manipulated through the psychophysical tools these practices provide, sometimes allowing the practitioner to perform feats that seem out of the range of normal human possibilities. At higher levels, they even allow the practitioner to experience a pure oneness with the universe (call it God, if you wish), without resorting to prayer, belief in a "personal God," or "salvation" as prerequisites for entry into eternal bliss, as is espoused by modern Christianity.

Chi power is not Satanic, demonic, or evil. It is part of the physical power spectrum naturally available to humans. This power is not invested in the body; it is a result of the very communications the body uses to function within itself and to interact with the world. To be anti-chi power is to be ignorant of the fact that without chi, you would die, not because chi is a substance that causes life or that fills some sort of vulnerable void, but because it is a manifestation of the body's physical operation. It is a flowing field that surrounds nerve impulses. It is, by definition, a natural condition of life that, like muscles, can be enhanced and put to practical use through development and will-power. Because an absence of chi indicates an absence of life, it is not something you want to be without. And further, demonizing it and the practices that foster its development is counterproductive to one's true spiritual advancement.

> The nature of God is a circle of which the center is everywhere and the circumference is nowhere
>
> —Empedocles

5. The Alchemy of Chi

Tai Chi Chuan is called a superior martial art, an excellent exercise, a mode of moving meditation, and a practice that enhances well-being on a deep level. Less has been said about its kinship to spiritual alchemy, but this last aspect is, perhaps, Tai Chi's most important gift to the practitioner.

The Taijitu and the CNS/ENS

To begin to understand how tai chi promotes spiritual alchemy, let's first look at the taijitu—the famous tai chi symbol—and its relationship to the physical mechanisms that enable the production of chi and, eventually, spiritual alchemy.

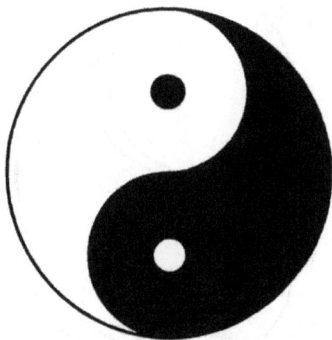

The taijitu normally is depicted as a static circle divided by a wavy line, with the area on one side of the line colored white and the other side colored black. (Figure 5.1) The larger portion of each side contains a spot of the opposite color. The two halves often are referred to as "fish," and the spots of color as "eyes." The bounding circle represents the totality of the universe—of reality. The white half, called yang, is indicative of energy, motion, or action, while the dark half, called yin, is the space or matter that energy impinges or acts upon, moves, or causes to act. The mutual interaction of the positive and negative forces of yang and

Figure 5.1 The taijitu depicts the major forces of opposition and cooperation that underlie the functioning of reality.

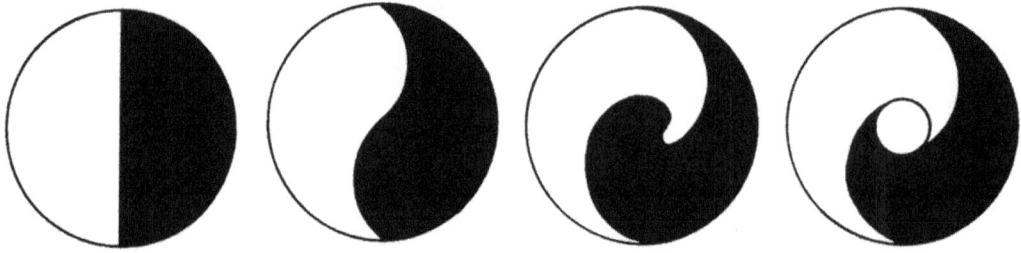

Figure 5.2 The tai chi symbol does not depict a static state but dynamic movement much like a spiral or vortex that spins around a central point.

yin—in differing strengths, amounts, and distribution—spawns the manifestations of multifold reality.

But the taijitu only seems to be static. In reality, it depicts a snapshot of motion, with the movement spinning clockwise, in the direction of the yang fish's head, round and round within the bounding circle. The greater the velocity of the spin of the two fishes, the more the spin will create a vortex at its center, much like hurricanes, tornados, or water going down a drain. (Figure 5.2) In a very real sense, this is similar to the idea in physics that you can observe energy as either a particle—a snapshot of how it would appear if it were motionless—or as a wave in motion, but not both simultaneously. The static taijitu is the static particle, the vortex the energy in motion.

Normally, the taijitu is depicted as in Figure 5.1, with the yang fish at the top, head to the right. But in reality, the spin can be reversed, with the yang fish's head pointing to the left and the spin revolving counter-clockwise. This reversal can be accomplished without halting the energy's momentum by threading the energy around the head of the yang fish then on past its tail. (Figure 5.3) If the spinning is thus reversed on every half spin, the wavy line forms a figure eight.

Although the Chinese who created the tai chi symbol could not know that an elongated figure eight laid on its side eventually would be used as a symbol for infinity, it is interesting that the infinity symbol

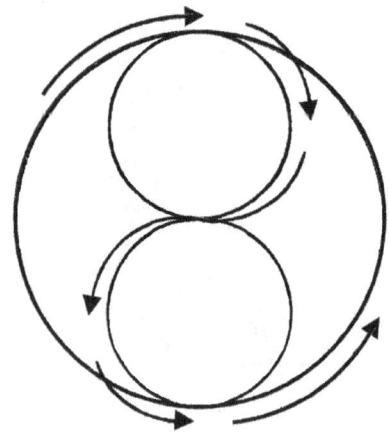

Figure 5.3 If the taijitu reverses on every other spin, it creates a figure eight.

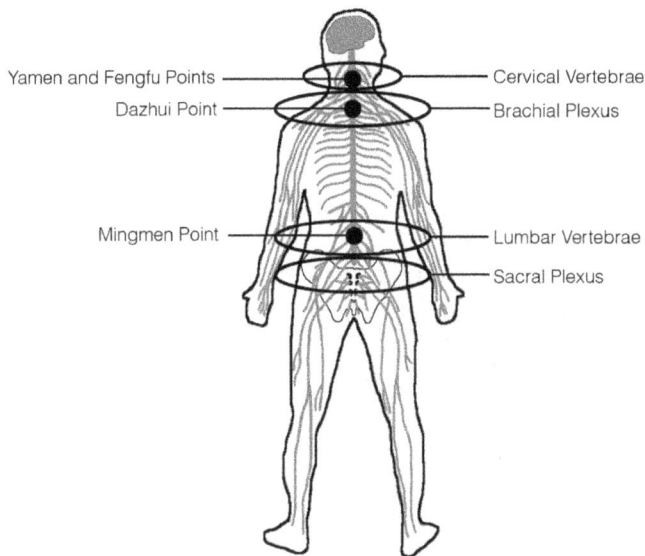

Figure 5.4 Important nerve plexus centers, spinal sections, and acupuncture points located along the Governing Vessel. Chi is channeled into the legs at the sacral plexus, and it is channeled into the arms at the brachial plexus.

crops up here within another symbol for the eternal void. Nor could they know that, centuries later, this figure eight also would depict an important aspect of Tai Chi Chuan: the constant twisting and reversing hip/waist motion of the Tai Chi Chuan exponent when viewed from above that is so important to the martial functioning of this art. What they must have known, however, was that the tai chi symbol describes something even more important: the two physiological structures that form the Microcosmic Orbit, which is the principal circuit for the creation and flow of chi within the body.

These two physiological structures are the Governing Vessel, which runs from the perineum, up the spine, and through the top of the head to the hard palate, and the Conception Vessel, which runs down through the front of the body to the perineum. As I show in my book, *The Wellspring: An Inquiry into the Nature of Chi*, chi is the flow or pulses of electromagnetism that accompany the sequential firing of electrical impulses or signals along nerves. The electrical flow or pulses are generated in a power center called the tantien, located in the area below and behind one's navel. Most of the flow is channeled upward through the spine and brain, while some of it is channeled into the limbs at nerve centers located along the spine: into the legs at a location that corresponds to the sacral plexus and into the arms at the brachial plexus. (Figure 5.4)

Most people understand that the combined elements of the Central Nervous System (CNS)—brain and spine—contain most of the body's nerves, but many do not realize that the intestines contain more neurons than the spine and entire rest of the body put together, not counting the brain. This places the major mass of this neural complex—called the Enteric Nervous System (ENS)—

right in the tantien. In short, the ENS undoubtedly *is* the tantien. Along with the esophagus and stomach, the ENS forms the Conception Vessel, which is the yin portion of the Microcosmic Orbit, while the spinal column and brain form the Governing Vessel, which is the yang portion. And again, chi flow is the electromagnetic flow or pulse that accompanies the flow of bioelectricity through the Microcosmic Orbit and the twelve additional chi channels—called meridians—that run through the arms and legs —three in each limb—in conjunction with the main nerves there. The totality of the chi "circulatory system" is referred to as the Macrocosmic Orbit.

At first glance, it's difficult to discern commonalities between the CNS and the ENS, but a little closer look reveals an important similarity: Both the brain and intestinal mass exhibit intensely convoluted folding of the tissues. The reason for this in both instances is to increase the surface area of these organs. In the case of the brain, it is believed that the folding increases brain power, while the extensive folding of the intestines, and especially its lining, increases the surface area available for the completion of digestion and the absorption of nutrients.[1]

All this folding makes these two major nerve centers bear an uncanny resemblance to one another, but perhaps more to the point is the fact that, when we regard ourselves as thinking beings, we tend to "feel" that the seat of our consciousness resides somewhere inside our heads—not at any specific location, perhaps, but at some locus that shifts position slightly within our heads depending on circumstance. Likewise, when practitioners of chi-en-

> The final result of long practice and proper execution of Tai-Chi Chuan comes into sight when the practitioner achieves an internal cleansing which is manifested as a clear flame or fire. This flame is the image of unity within the individual, resulting from disengagement from the confusing and distracting physical surroundings. Eventually, while practicing Tai-Chi Chuan time and space are no longer relevant. The practitioner does not even perceive the presence of other people. Neither sight, sound, nor the passing of time pierce concentration of the Tai-Chi Chuan. When this stage occurs, one is no longer a separate unity but mixes with the universe and becomes reconnected to the unity of everything. One has progressed from achieving personal unity, the first great achievement in the practice of Tai-Chi Chuan, to the next step of identification with the universe. Thus the environment of the fourth dimension is near.
>
> —Jou Tsung Hwa
> *The Tao of Tai-Chi Chuan*

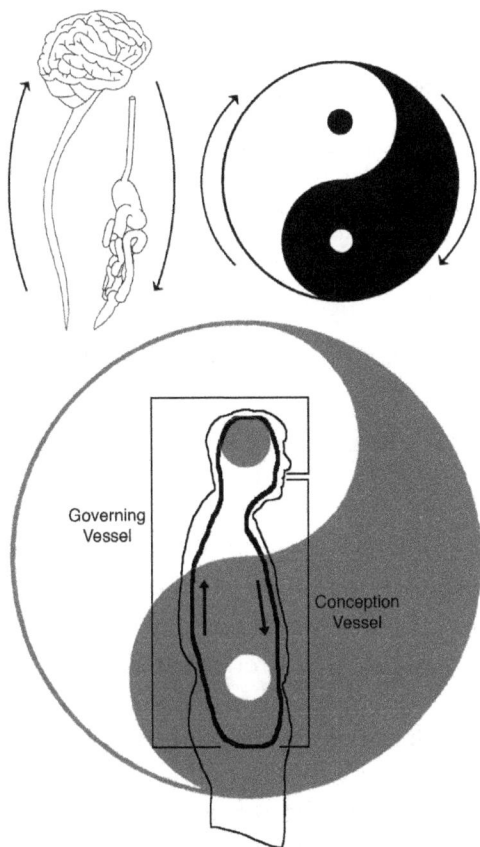

Figure 5.5 There is an amazing correspondence between the tai chi symbol and the composite physiological elements of the Microcosmic Orbit, including similarities in appearance, orientation, and direction of energy flow.

hancing exercises experience themselves as motile beings, they tend to "feel" that the seat of their chi resides in an equally nonspecific but centralized locus within the mass of their gut. After all, the iconic image of the master meditating on his navel isn't an amusing aspersion to one who understands that the navel is the slightly off-center bull's-eye of the tantien.

If we map the circuit of the taijitu onto the circuit of the microcosmic orbit, their relative shapes and positions give us a very interesting visual image. (Figure 5.5) The CNS is a mass (brain) with a tail that descends (spine), while the ENS is a mass (entrails) with a tail that ascends (stomach and esophagus). Together they form a sort of rough tai chi symbol that is properly displayed, with the body of the yang fish (CNS) at the top and the body of the yin fish (ENS) at the bottom. Or rather, it is the tai chi symbol that is properly drawn and oriented to depict the physiological structure of the Microcosmic Orbit.

Add the idea of spinning, and the symbol actually depicts the chi flowing through the Microcosmic Orbit in the proper direction. In addition, the fishes' eyes can be seen as symbolic of the physiological attachment of the tail end of each fish—or nerve center—within the mass of the opposite fish: the tongue touching the hard palate and the tailbone connecting with the end of the intestinal tract through the intervening tissue of the perineum. Or, the eyes could symbolize the seed of awareness within each fish of the existence of the other. In any case, nothing is ever completely and totally yin or yang—at least not within the reality in which we live and within which everything is relative.

> The New Testament teaches dying to one's self, literally suffering the pain of death to the world and its values. This is the vocabulary of the mystics. Now, suicide is also a symbolic act. It casts off the psychological posture that you happen to be in at the time, so that you may come into a better one. You die to your current life in order to come to another of some kind. But, as Jung says, you'd better not get caught in a symbolic situation. You don't have to die, really, physically. All you have to do is die spiritually and be reborn to a larger way of living.
>
> —Joseph Campbell
> *The Power of Myth*

The visual similarity between the physiological constructs of the central and enteric nervous systems and the yang and yin fish of the tai chi symbol is too remarkable to be coincidence. The creators of the tai chi symbol must have drawn it as a sort of esoteric guidepost to help initiates who seek to strengthen and mobilize their chi. In this, they were in line with a tradition in the West that arose completely separately but that had similar aims in mind: alchemy. And indeed, some of the precepts and practices of both arts overlap, and both frequently resort to symbolic representation to transmit their truths—symbolic representations that often have been distorted by those unaware of their true import.

Alchemy

Ultimately, chi enhancing exercises can be thought of as true alchemy. That is, in addition to being physical and mental disciplines, chi-enhancing exercises also are part of a more esoteric practice designed to induce spiritual awakening.

Most people look on the alchemist as a primitive chemist who attempted to distill a concoction of sulfur and mercury to create either gold or the fabled Philosopher's Stone—a substance believed to have the power to transmute base metals into gold or, in some traditions, that could be consumed like a drug to achieve enlightenment. Although true alchemy does have the goals of spiritual awakening and symbolic immortality, contrary to these popular misconceptions, true alchemy has nothing to do with metal, and even less with chemistry, and it does not produce a pill that can be consumed.

Instead, the various elements, metals, and processes are really metaphors behind which ancient alchemists hid the truth of their research and methods, either out of fear of religious persecution or to keep the secrets of true spiritual

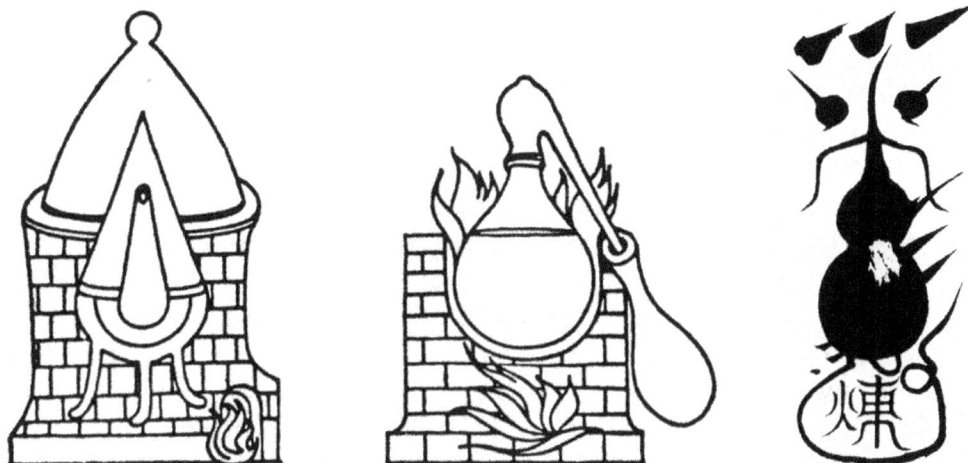

Figure 5.6 Athanors of classical Western alchemy (left and center) and the Talisman of the Ruler of the South (right), an ancient Taoist symbol used in refining spiritual energy. The similarities are remarkable.

power hidden from the unworthy and corrupt. Later men, ignorant of the allegorical and metaphorical nature of the descriptions, took them as literal recipes and techniques and attempted to use them to transmute lead into gold, eventually developing the modern science of chemistry.

The classical description of alchemical work is that the alchemist mixes mercury and sulfur in a retort called an alembic or athanor (Figure 5.6), and repeatedly heats and cools the sulfur and mercury mixture with a fire underneath. After enough cooking and cooling, the refined result rises up the spout of the retort and is emitted as gold or as the Philosopher's Stone. From the viewpoint of modern chemistry, this description is ludicrous despite the fact that its misguided founders did their best to achieve these results.

Looking past the surface, however, the description begins to make sense. Sulfur is symbolic of the spirit, or active aspect of nature, while mercury is symbolic of the soul, or passive aspect of nature—the yang and yin. They also signify the Governing and Conception Vessels, respectively. These two aspects of nature and their major energy channels generally are present within the human being in an unrefined and separated state. However, when the mind and breath are concentrated in the tantien, as with the abdominal breathing techniques of meditation and chi-enhancing exercises such as chi kung or Tai Chi, a heat is produced in the body that is both physical and psychic. This is the fire, and the abdominal area—the tantien—is the retort or athanor in which one refines the active and passive aspects of one's being. The gold or Philosopher's

Stone that is the refined product of alchemy is not a precious metal or a pill, and the base metal from which the gold is transmuted is not lead. Instead, the gold is enlightenment, transmuted from base nature.

Over time, with continual practice, development of the tantien produces a heat that is both physical and psychic and that acts to refine and condense the conflicting aspects—the yang and yin—within the human being into a unified whole, producing a more powerful chi flow. Little by little, as the chi strengthens and its flow through the Microcosmic Orbit increases, coalesces, and comes under conscious control, its powerful pressure can be encouraged to rise through the Governing Vessel, which is the spout of the retort, opening the chakras, or power centers along the spine, as it rises. The sequential opening of the chakras enables or activates a form of energy that is higher than chi—spiritual energy. This spiritual energy also circulates through the Microcosmic Orbit along with the chi, and eventually, it fountains out of its bounding circuit through the crown chakra (the fontanel, or, Thousand Petal Lotus), linking one directly with Creation and resulting in enlightenment.

So chi-enhancing exercises are, essentially, methods of achieving health and well-being through refinement of body, awareness, and will by means of particular physical exercises that use the mechanism of abdominal breathing to strengthen and mobilize the chi and to induce and empower spiritual energy, hopefully leading not only to physical well-being and personal empowerment, but to higher states of consciousness.

Pure alchemy in a run-on sentence.

Excerpted in part from:
The Wellspring: An Inquiry into the Nature of Chi
(Phosphene Publishing Co., 2008)

6. Auras

There are rare individuals who claim they can see auras of light surrounding other people. Skeptics scoff at such a notion, but perhaps we can look at the phenomenon with Tai Chi eyes. Auras are usually described as egg-shaped energy fields that surround the human body that manifest visually in various colors dependent on the psyche and personality of the individual. So, there are two questions: 1) Does the human body produce an energy field? and 2) If so, is it possible that such an energy field can be detected by some human eyes?

Regarding the possible existence of such fields, the fact is that the human body is a biological electrical generator, and nerve impulses are nothing more than a flow of bioelectricity—in the form of ions—along the nerves. The major flow of nerve impulses occurs along the spine, in the brain, and through the Enteric Plexus located within the digestive system, which contains more neurons than the entire rest of the nervous system, including the spine but not the brain. The flow of energy through these structures forms a loop, or complete circuit, inside the torso and head—a loop known as the Microcosmic Orbit. Any electrical source produces an electrical field around itself, and electricity that moves along a conductor or through a complete circuit also produces an electromagnetic field that flows perpendicularly around the axis of the current. Therefore, there must be an electrical/electromagnetic field that surrounds the human body, and such a field will be egg-shaped rather than spherical due to deformation caused by Earth's gravity, which affects magnetic and electromagnetic fields as much as it does matter.

Another scientific fact is that any energetic action that excites electrons, which are the basic components of electricity, casts out photons, or light, even if most of us can't see it without special equipment. Infrared light, for example, emanates at frequencies that are too low to be seen by the average human eye, but it can be registered by infrared cameras or goggles. Ultraviolet light, which lies along the electromagnetic spectrum above the average threshold of sight, also can be made visible via special equipment. More sophisticated equipment can detect X-rays, gamma rays, and other even more energetic portions of the electromagnetic spectrum.

Many animals, however, have natural visual structures that allow them to see farther into either of the extremes of infrared or ultraviolet than humans can. Often this is associated with night vision, as with cats and various nocturnal animals. And as we all know, while we might prefer to treat all people with equal respect and opportunity, humans have a wide variety of characteristics, not all of which are equal in all people. Some people have smarter brains, some have stronger muscles, some hear more acutely, and others see more sharply.

But the human eye is not simply a telescope that functions better in some than in others. It is a complex structure whose components, such as the photoreceptor cells that gather incoming photons and translate them into nerve signals, while generally adhering to a basic blueprint, actually have a range of weaknesses and strengths. Some people, for example, see sharply enough but are colorblind to one or more frequencies of light and cannot see the full range of color available to the average person. Such people are at the low end of the spectrum of color perception. Likewise, there undoubtedly are people whose range of color perception extends beyond that of the average person, either into the infrared or the ultraviolet. Some artists, for example, have been noted for their sensitivity to ranges of color most of us can't identify or define. It is possible, then, that such people might be able to perceive frequencies of light emanating from the energy fields—auras—surrounding other people that the rest of us can't see.

It would be interesting to listen to a description of a Tai Chi master performing peng, say, from a person with the ability to perceive auras. How would the Tai Chi master's field alter—in shape, color, or other characteristic—during the gathering and expulsion of internal chi energy that peng entails? Or how would the field of a chi kung master whose powerful chi is in full circulation and whose field is strong—appear to a person who can see auras?

While auras apparently can be visually perceived by some people, the true nature of auras is often misunderstood by people who have heard about them but who can't perceive them directly. Much Christian religious imagery, for example, shows saints with halos floating just above their heads. These halos are simplistic depictions of the extraordinarily powerful auras projected by such people as interpreted by artists and others ignorant of the nature and presence of these biological fields, which surround the entire body, not just the crown of the head. It is perhaps true, though, that a person's aura is more powerful at the crown of the head. That is close to the prominent electromagnetic field of the brain, and the fontanel is reputed to be the place that can "open" to allow one's spirit to merge with the universal consciousness.

Furthermore auras aren't just visual. For those of us whose eyes function within the average range of color perception, they can be perceived in other ways. In Tai Chi, it is said that a master can sense changes in an opponent's field and react accordingly, even before the opponent has moved. It is said that such a master can "feel" the opponent with his skin. The skin—and particularly the hairs protruding from it—is the first tangible layer that exists between a Tai Chi Chuanist and his opponent. And if chi is principally the internal flow of the body's electromagnetic energy and the field that is subsequently produced around the body, it makes perfect sense that the hairs would be sensitized by alterations in an opponent's field since bodily hairs are sensitive to electromagnetic fields and charges—think of how a static electrical charge can raise the hairs on your arm or head and prickle the skin beneath.

Tai Chi, chi kung, and other chi-based exercises work to relax the body enough to allow the practitioner to feel the flow within, and the more this occurs, the more sensitive the practitioner becomes to the sensation of external fields impinging upon the practitioner's own body and field. In fact, Tai Chi's dynamics include both physical and energetic movements that operate in conjunction. The practice increases the output of the body's field, and the movements of the limbs act to create swirls, whirlpools, and waves within the practitioner's own field and within the field of the opponent, as well.

Yang–Yin

A Chinese symbol of the dual distribution of forces, comprising the active or masculine principle (Yang) and the passive or feminine principle (Yin). It takes the form of a circle bisected by a sigmoid line, and the two parts so formed are invested with a dynamic tendency which would be wanting if the division were by a diameter. The light half represents the Yang force and the dark half denotes Yin; however, each half includes an arc cut out of the middle of the opposing half, to symbolize that every mode must contain within it the germ of its antithesis. Guénon considers that the Yang–Yin is a helicoidal symbol, that is, that it is a section of the universal whirlwind which brings opposites together and engenders perpetual motion, metamorphosis, and continuity in situations characterized by contradiction. The entrance to and exit from this movement lie outside the movement itself, in the same way that birth and death stand apart from the life of the individual in so far as it is conscious and self-determined. The vertical axis through the centre of the Yang–Yin constitutes the "unvarying mean," or, in other words, the mystic "Centre" where there is no rotation, no restlessness, no impulse, nor any suffering of any kind. It corresponds to the central zone of the Wheel of Transformations in Hindu symbolism, and the centre or the way out of the labyrinth in Egyptian and western symbolism. It is also expressive of the two counter balancing tendencies of evolution and involution.

—J.E. Cirlot
A Dictionary of Symbols

Part III

Tai Chi that Isn't Tai Chi but Is Tai Chi

7. Introduction

Tai Chi concepts and literature are filled with dichotomy. We often see statements like: "If there is up, there is down," or "Defense and attack are simultaneous." But dichotomy in Tai Chi should come as no surprise. The art is based on yin/yang, and it's name is derived from Taoist/Buddhist principles and from the tai chi symbol—the taijitu—which is a profound and universally recognized representation of all dichotomies.

The title of this section might seem to indicate that my subject is dichotomies, and perhaps it is in the final reckoning. But after a time, as implied by the second statement above, such dichotomies tend to coalesce into unified wholes that contain both the yin and yang in different mixtures. So, drawing a particular yin/yang analogy isn't my purpose here. Instead, I want to talk about the whole of the mutual interaction between Tai Chi and living in the phenomenal world.

When I first came to Tai Chi, I was looking for a martial art that would exercise my body and impart some measure of self-defense ability. Above all, I wanted it to be interesting enough to absorb me for some time. Little did I realize that "some time" meant "a lifetime." Nor did I realize just how deeply my Tai Chi practice would affect my interactions with the phenomenal world.

As the movements and energies of Tai Chi have become more and more integrated into my body, I find myself moving through life in a tai chi way, not only physically but intellectually and emotionally. I can see how practice of Tai Chi and adherence to its principles smoothes one's experiences and how lack of adherence enables or creates turmoil. Now, more than four decades later, I understand that tai chi has much to impart beyond acquiring a more or less profound kinetic sense and developing and manipulating internal energy—and by extension, developing the ability to manipulate the kinetic senses and energies of others.

But the ways that Tai Chi connects the Tai Chi player with the world is only half of the story. The other half is how the world constantly connects back, demonstrating Tai Chi principles in ways ranging from subtle to obvious. The longer I've practiced, the more it seems that reality itself constantly manifests the principles of the art and delivers Tai Chi lessons at every turn. We just have to become aware of those lessons. And the interesting thing is that they often aren't always directly connected to the art—hence the title of this series.

"Tai Chi that Isn't Tai Chi that Is Tai Chi" features short pieces on some of the lessons I've learned over the years from incidents and other means and sources that weren't specifically Tai Chi-related but that perfectly exhibit or demonstrate some element of the art. I have to admit here, that I basically stole the idea for the title from the subtitle of William Ting's *Essential Concepts of Tai Chi: It is – It is Not – IT IS*.[1] But as I pointed out in my review of that excellent book, it's pretty much what Bruce Lee said about the concept of the punch.

I took up Tai Chi in my late twenties, so I'd had ample opportunity before that to experience life BTC (Before Tai Chi), and in retrospect, some of what I experienced seems to me now to have been specific lessons to prepare me for learning the art I've come to love and depend on. And since then, I have seen or experienced many similar lessons. They've helped me delve more deeply into Tai Chi, and I hope they do something similar for you.

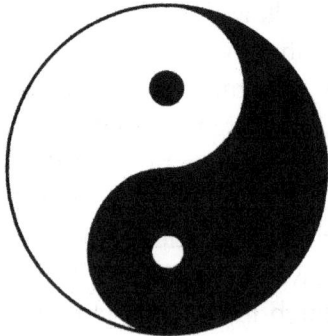

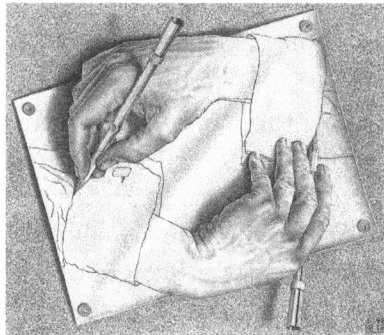

2

8. Oaken Limbs

A lot of readers might be familiar with the parable of the oak tree and the willow that grew next to it. For many seasons, the oak grew tall and extended strong branches, while the willow, with its drooping boughs, seemed weak in comparison. In fact, through the years, the oak frequently disparaged the willow, much like jocks bully nerds. But then came a reckoning in the form of a terrible storm whose winds relentlessly battered the two trees. Finally, a succession of terrific gusts uprooted the oak, which crashed to the ground beside the willow. The willow, however, with its supple branches, was still standing when the storm subsided.

The parable might have something to say about braggadocio and payback, so maybe the oak should have knocked on wood when it was boasting about its strength. But the parable is really about the ability to provide the least resistance possible when confronted with a seemingly overwhelming force—a Tai Chi maxim. However, when talking about Tai Chi, the oak tree isn't always the fall guy.

I had an interesting lesson in Tai Chi about six years before I ever heard of the art. I was in Austin at the time, visiting a friend, and one afternoon, we walked from his garage apartment to a nearby park to hang out. For a time, I lay on my back beneath an oak tree, with the crown of my head nearly touching the base of the trunk, which was about three feet in diameter. As I lay there, a gusty breeze was blowing through the tree branches, and I observed something I'd never noticed. I guess I'd always thought of wind rustling the leaves of trees or causing the branches to wave if the wind was strong enough, but my prone perspective of this tree showed a new dimension of behavior.

The breeze was strong enough to shake the limbs, but they did not simply move independently of the trunk —as if the trunk was a rigid pole and the limbs were just moving back and forth. Instead, as the force of the breeze impacted the broad, if irregular, surfaces of the foliage, several branches in any given area would flex in unison. And it wasn't only the branches that were flexing. The trunk was twisting slightly back and forth with

> Be careful, however, not to think of the tree as being stiff or rigid. Your neck, for example, though in line with your head and torso, must always be freely movable, ready to turn in any direction, left, right, or way around. It cannot swivel easily as required to by the instructions if there is any tautness in it. Waist movements are also of the utmost importance, and there should be no rigidity to prevent you from turning at the waist.
>
> —Edward Maisel
> *Tai Chi for Health*

the flexing branches, around its central core. Maybe for the first time, I saw a tree as a real living being, though not all trees can flex and twist in this manner, only straight-trunked one with sufficiently balanced branches. Tall, spindly tress probably just sway, and brushy trash trees probably just thrash. But then, neither type has as well-developed a central equilibrium as does a straight-trunked oak.

Many years later, when I finally loosened my waist, torso, and shoulders enough to open my body to the twisting of the trunk of my body around its central equilibrium, with the arms flexibly following the movement, I recalled not only the lesson this oak had taught me, but also a popular dance from the early 1960s called the Twist, which I'll cover in the next chapter.

> When someone tosses you a tea bowl
> —Catch it!
> Catch it nimbly with soft cotton
> With the cotton of your skillful mind
>
> —Bankei

9. The Twist

From 1959 to about 1965, a dance craze called the Twist took over dance floors all across the country. I was a tween during part of that time, and I was soon Twisting along with everybody else.

Words can't really describe the Twist, but here's the *Wikipedia* entry on how the Twist is performed:

> The twist is performed by standing with the feet approximately shoulder width apart. The torso may be squared to the knees and hips, or turned at an angle so one foot is farther forward than the other. The arms are held out from the body, bent at the elbow. The hips, torso, and legs rotate on the balls of the feet as a single unit, with the arms staying more or less stationary. The feet grind back and forth on the floor, and the dance can be varied in speed, intensity, and vertical height as necessary. Occasionally one leg is lifted off the floor for styling, but generally the dance posture is low and with the feet in contact with the floor with very little vertical motion.[1]

To really get the idea, go to *YouTube* and call up a video of Chubby Checker or other people Twisting. If you do, you'll see that the Twist requires one to use alternating pushes from the legs to twist the waist and hips back and forth. The waist is flexibly connected through the torso to the shoulders, which also twists back and forth, but alternating with the twisting of the hips and waist. The twisting of the waist and torso then propels the arms forward and backward. Above this movement, the head is held steady, as if suspended from above. And through it all, the body rotates around its central axis, though often not neatly. This was, after all, a flamboyant dance, not Tai Chi.

But the combined actions of the Twist are very similar to the way the legs, hips/waist, torso, shoulders, and head move around Central Equilibrium during Tai Chi. Of course there are differences, too. In the Twist, the feet make no attempt to root, there is some leaning of the torso, and many of the body movements are flashier than you'd find in Tai Chi. And more limited. But the principles of the dance are remarkably similar to the principles of Tai Chi.

Considering the timing of the dance with the advent of Tai Chi in the United States in the late 1950s, one might be tempted to think that the art

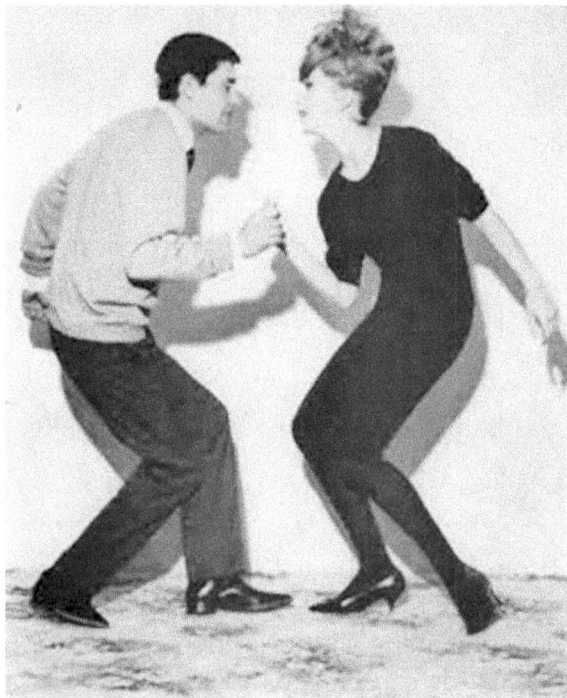

1

somehow spawned the dance, but that's not the case. The dance has roots that go back to the nineteenth century. In their book, *Jazz Dance*, Marshall and Jean Stearns state that a pelvic dance motion called the Twist came to America from the Congo during slavery.[2]

The alternation of life and death, condensation and dissolution, the predominance of Yang or of Yin, are, for the Taoist, like the alternating "waves" of thread in the weave of a fabric.

—J.E. Cirlot
A Dictionary of Symbols

72

10. The Waist Is the Commander

The statement, "The waist is the commander," is familiar to most Tai Chi exponents above the level of beginner. The hips and waist comprise the mechanism that transfers and directs the energy surging up from the legs into the correct upper body part in the correct manner. The following incident might or might not illustrate that point, but it showed me how action of the abdominal region can instinctively initiate and control movement.

I was about ten years old at the time, living in central Oklahoma. At the end of the road I lived on was a large, wooded tract of property owned by a widow and her son. A prominent creek ran along the back line of the property, and my friends and I liked to explore the creek and the property itself, which had several features of interest to mischievous boys, such as a forest fire watchtower, a large hay barn, and a small brick gazebo built like a guard house into one corner of the tall brick wall that formed the front property line.

Eventually, someone had the idea that there was oil underneath the property. The surrounding neighborhoods notwithstanding, an oil exploration crew moved in, drilled an exploratory well, and generally trashed and spoiled the back third of the property before discovering that only dirt and rock lay beneath. The exploration company moved on, leaving a huge, muddy scar on the landscape, including two highly polluted detention ponds colored an iridescent vomit green. These ponds lay just slightly uphill and less than a quarter of a mile from the creek. It was just the sort of place for my friend, John, and I to explore. And others, too.

One day, John and I were down there, at the back side of the lowest detention pond, where a fringe of woods separated the "oil field" from the creek. As we were messing around, a couple of girls about our age or a little older showed up from the woods. I'd never seen them before, so they were probably from one of the new neighborhoods that were being developed on the far side of the creek. Apparently, they didn't like the fact that my friend and I were there, so they started throwing rocks at us.

Well, I'd been in plenty of rock, dirt clod, and walnut battles, and I wasn't intimidated. I picked up some missiles of my own and threw back. Both pairs of us hunkered down behind mounds of dirt about thirty feet apart, then we'd pop up and give fire before ducking down again, with lots of grade-school curse words hurled in between. After this had gone on for maybe five minutes, I popped up to throw another rock, and was greeted with an odd sight.

One of the girls had risen above her protective mound, and I could see her clearly from about mid thigh up—except for a weird black patch that blocked much of her upper torso. This black patch was very irregular in shape, kind like an elongated and twisted blob with half a dozen spindly and raggedly sharp projections jutting from its main body. It seemed to be hanging mysteriously in the air between me and the girl, whose arm was weirdly extended toward me.

In the split second that I saw the blob, my mind reacted, trying to figure out what it was. "Root," a voice proclaimed. "She just threw it. It's flying right at your head!"

All that information came as if in one instantaneous word. I felt a seed of panic appear inside me. The piece of root with the jagged remains of smaller roots sticking out of it, was going to hit me right in the face. But the panic had no chance to sprout. In that instant, I felt muscles wrench inside my lower abdomen, jerking me downward with a speed that I could never have accomplished consciously. As my body contracted, I felt the root tips graze the top of my head as the ragged chunk sailed over me. I'd been saved by my tantien, which had reacted to the danger even before my conscious mind had recognized it.

> Stillness in the heart of movement
> is the secret of all power.
>
> —John Blofeld
> *Taoist Mysteries and Magic*

11. AirDancers

Who'd have thought they actually have a name? AirDancers. But of course, they are signs, and their designers probably couldn't help but give them designations.

AirDancers (Figure 11.1) are those flexible, fan-inflated, Gumby-like figures that you see in front of used car dealerships, strip malls, and other businesses. The fan blows air up through the tube of the torso, and the air whips the arms as it surges through them before being released at the hands.

Sound familiar? In the case of Air-Dancers, the energy that is propelled upward is air, while in the case of Tai Chi Chuanists, the energy is chi, but it's interesting that the force that moves upward in both cases does so in pulses that originate at the bottom, in the feet/fan. In addition, it doesn't just push upward. Instead, it moves in a corkscrew pattern. In the case of the AirDancer, energy is propelled upward through the tube body by the screwing motion of the fan blades, while in the case of the Tai Chi Chuanist, it's chi that is twisted down the legs to the feet, resurged into the legs, and twisted back

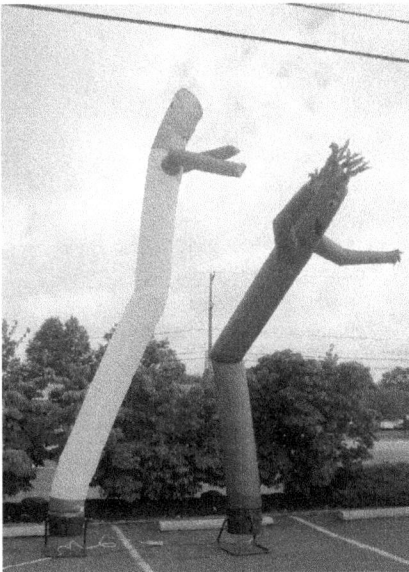

Figure 11.1 AirDancers sparring.[1]

upward into the torso. The torso continues the twisting, which whips the arms, the force terminating in the hands.

So the mechanism of both is roughly the same—both employing an upward twisting of energy that also is linked in both to "air." I'd bet that one of those AirDancers, though completely devoid of strength—or even real substance— could give you a pretty good whack if you happened to be in range of one of its whipping hands.

Sure sounds like Tai Chi.

Floating with the Waves

There is a chi kung movement called Floating with the Waves. It is essentially performing Open Tai Chi over and over for a given number of repetitions. Imagine that you are at the beach, standing chest deep in the water just past the breakers, where the swells rise and fall in peaceful, rhythmic waves. Your arms are extended in front of you, lying relaxed on the surface of the water as you face the open ocean. As each swell surges in and out, it will buoy your arms and body up then lower them down.

In the early 1970s, I was married to a woman who had an amazing ability to float effortlessly on those same sorts of swells. We'd swim out there, and she'd just float on her back, totally at ease and at one with the water. As for me, I could float for only a very short time before my legs and arms began to drag me down.

She was a water sign—a Cancer—so maybe that had something to do with her affinity with the ocean. Also, she was born on the Gulf Coast and had been playing in these waters since she was a child. More likely, though, her body mass index almost perfectly equalled that of sea water. Whatever the reason, she could lie there as long as she wanted, expending absolutely no energy, yet riding the variations of energy waves coming her way with perfect ease. So blended was she within her element that it seemed to me as if her body almost magically rippled along with the water, mimicking every tiny variation in its flow.

She, of course, thought nothing of it, for it was totally effortless on her part.

12. Tesla's Oscillator

Nicola Tesla was one of the world's greatest inventors and innovators. We owe much of our current state of technology to him—pun intended. He invented, among other things, the AC electric generator, the AC motor, radio remote control, florescent lighting, and the loudspeaker. His patents for radio transmission were used illicitly by Guglielmo Marconi in the latter's "invention" of the radio, and that fact was eventually recognized by the U.S. Patent Office, which upheld Tesla's rights to the technology, though this judgment occurred after Tesla's death. He also attempted but failed to use the idea of transmission of radio waves to transmit electrical power without wires, and he purportedly invented a "death ray" that utilized similar technology.

More to the point of Tai Chi, Tesla was fascinated by oscillation—both wave motion and vibration—not just on an energetic level, as with radio transmission, but on a mechanical level. The following story about Tesla is apocryphal. Some insist it actually happened, while others say it is just a tall tale told about this wizard of science. But Tai Chi folks might readily recognize the possibilities.

At the time, Tesla's laboratory was located on the sixth floor of a building in New York City. Once day, people from the neighborhood around the building began flocking to the local police station, complaining that an earthquake was shaking their homes. The supposed earthquake could not be felt at the police station, but because of the number of complaints and the sincerity of the witnesses, the police chief went out with a team of officers to investigate.

Sure enough, as the police entered the neighborhood, they felt the ground shaking and saw the effects of the movement on the surrounding buildings. The deeper they went into the neighborhood, the greater the shaking became. The chief then realized that Tesla's lab was located at the quake's epicenter, and he and his men entered the building, where the shaking was almost nonexistent. They rushed up the stairs and burst into the lab. As they did, the chief saw Tesla raise a heavy hammer and smash it down on a small box affixed to a steel support pillar. The shaking immediately stopped.

Supposedly, Tesla had been researching mechanical oscillation and had devised a small wave-effect oscillator that sent a tiny but rhythmic pounding against the support pillar. This pillar was fastened solidly to the New York City bedrock, and over time, the oscillations created by his device, minute though they were, set up a series of ever amplified waveforms. These eventually began to oscillate the bedrock, which in turn, sent concentric waves through the ground, outward from the building, mimicking an earthquake. When Tesla smashed the device, the oscillations—and the earthquake—halted.

This story is, as I said, apocryphal, but on one level, it illustrates energy propagating outward from a solid center grounded with single-weightedness: the steel support pillar fastened to the bedrock. It also shows how relatively small inputs of energy properly amplified, channeled, and applied can have wide-ranging and damaging effects. And on yet a third tack, I once saw a demonstration by T. T. Liang that achieved the same effect in miniature, and I've heard that other masters have the same ability.

Liang, who was then in his mid nineties and using a cane, was accompanied by his chief student, Stuart Olson. Liang stood next to Olson, placed his palm on Olson's abdomen, and started vibrating his hand. In just a few seconds, Olson was vibrating, too, and after the vibrations built up over several seconds, Olson was forced to fall over backward.

I like to think that the Tesla story is genuine, but I know that Liang could utilize the same sort of effect on another person because I witnessed it. Good thing that Olson wasn't firmly fastened to the floor or maybe the whole auditorium eventually would have shaken!

Vibration techniques are called dou jin in Chinese. In bagua, with these techniques, the entire chi of the body is made to vibrate, which causes the opening and closing actions of the body to oscillate at high speed. This creates a machine-gun effect in which the opponent is hit with five or six full-power vibrating strikes in the blink of an eye.

—Bruce Frantzis
The Power of the Internal Martial Arts and Chi

13. Tai Chi in the Driveway

Tai Chi metaphors abound in reality. I guess that's because Tai Chi so closely adheres to natural laws. But you can find Tai Chi in a lot of things. One of them is sitting out in my driveway right now. My car. (Figure 13.1)

In Tai Chi, we can consider the legs to be the engine, the pelvic area to be the driver, and the torso and arms to be the car. This matches Tai Chi theory, which states that martial power is generated in the legs, directed by the waist, and manifested in the arms and hands. In a car, the raw energy from the engine is controlled and directed by the driver (ultimately by the driver's mind manifesting through physical movement to steer and use the pedals), and the car responds appropriately.

We can carry the Tai Chi/automobile analogy in a couple of other directions. First, it's kind of interesting that a driver generally uses a wheel to control and direct a vehicle, just as the Tai Chi Chuanist uses a wheel-like turning of the pelvic area to control and direct martial force and power. And in both cases, the main wheel turns other wheels to produce a dynamic effect, such as swerving to avoid an impact. In both car and Tai Chi, all movements are circular, and even sharp turns take curving paths, and in both, the navel always points straight ahead.

Second, controlling direction and angle of movement is only part of Tai Chi's martial aspect. There also is controlling the wave of internal energy that bolsters or is added to the movements, the sudden release of which is called fa jing. Similar in a car is using the gas pedal to send the car forward with a surge of acceleration or the brakes to suddenly withdraw. Ironically, both are performed while the driver is in a sitting posture and are done with a single foot—single-weightedness—and usually the Bubbling Well is just about where the pressure is applied to the pedals by the foot. And the movements that the two pedals cause alternate with one another, acceleration followed by braking followed by acceleration—yang followed by yin followed by yang—until the car returns to its parking spot and re-achieves the state of wu wei that it was in before you got in and drove it to the store, disturbing its equilibrium.

Furthermore, we all know that it isn't the flash of a car's exterior that makes a superior machine but what's under the hood. Its power plant. Its chi generator. And the mind of the driver has a great deal to do with how well the car (body) is utilized. An inexperienced or lousy

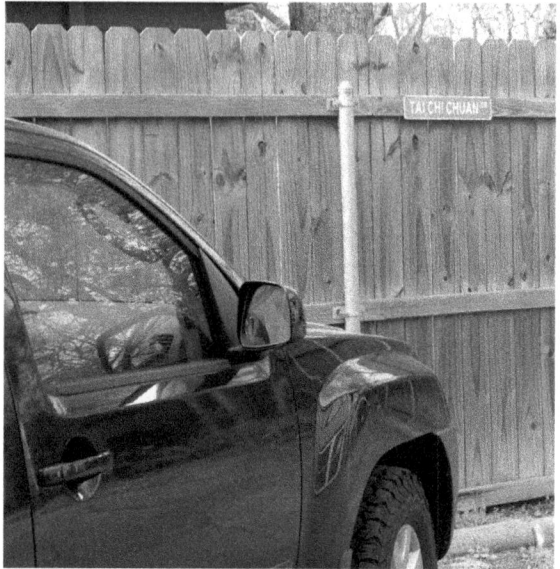

Figure 13.1 My car, like me, is a little beat up, but it's still headed down Tai Chi Chuan Drive.

driver will not drive as well as a seasoned and responsible driver, much less a pro, no matter what he's driving. So, just as in Tai Chi, the quality of the driver's intent and control are more important than the flash of the car's exterior or even the power under the hood. Though the latter certainly makes things better, ultimately, the best drivers are those for whom the car becomes an extension of the body, just as it is said that weapons, such as swords and spears, become extensions of the warrior. Ideally in both cases, the person thinks the thought of movement, and the extension follows that thought through a successive chain of actions that align perfectly to produce an aggregate result.

And just as with driving, the process of Tai Chi becomes automatic, most often occurring without conscious thought. If you're like most drivers, you've experienced the awakening that occurs after driving for some time then suddenly realizing you don't remember a thing about the last ten minutes. The awakening is because you're thankful to still be alive. Thank goodness your instinctual mind was in control, because your conscious mind sure wasn't! Tai Chi is similar in that if you use it without thinking, you're probably just as thankful.

If the engine is the power plant of the car (its generator of force and chi), we also need a way for that power to be manipulated to affect acceleration and

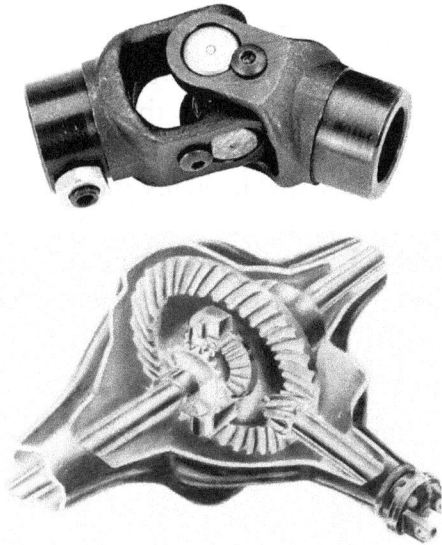

Figure 13.2 The mechanical transmission of power in a car requires a universal joint (top) and a differential gear (bottom). The former provides a flexible connection to transfer rotational energy from one shaft to another, and it functions similarly to the connection between the pelvis and the spine. The latter transfers rotational energy from a drive shaft to two axles that are at right angles to the drive shaft, and it functions similarly to the connections of the hips to both spine and legs.[1,2]

drive the wheels (the feet). That manipulation is accomplished by a combination of a universal joint (U-joint) and a differential gear. (Figure 13.2) The former provides a flexible connection from one drive shaft to another—such as from the pelvic area to the torso—and the latter is a gear device that can transfer rotational energy from one drive shaft (the spine) to two axles (hips/legs) that are at right angles to the drive shaft. This is the same kind of U-joint and differential gear arrangement that comprises the waist and hips, only in the case of the body, the feet torque the spine, torso, and ultimately arms through the differential gear and U-joint instead of the other way around.

Also, in addition to using mind to direct the vehicle or body, the driver and Tai Chi Chuanist both must possess an open sort of awareness that takes in one's surroundings without specific focus. With driving, we look ahead, out the side windows, and in our rearview mirrors with a constantly shifting gaze that tends to soft-focus in the middle distance when not briefly pausing on specific targets. Our ears are attuned for any of dozens of sounds that could signal a problem or crisis. Our noses are all too aware of the odors of burned rubber, oil, and that cloud of incompletely combusted gasoline from the car ahead that you were just forced to inhale. And through the steering wheel, our hands register the contours of the road beneath. These all are just as the Tai Chi Chuanist "listens" with his or her skin—and every other organ of perception—to the energy of the opponent and situation.

And finally, both Tai Chi and driving are dynamic undertakings with a few rules in common. First is to be rooted. As drivers, we all know not to uproot our vehicles by leaning them too far one way or another, particularly right in the middle of a dynamic maneuver, or by starting or stopping too fast. If you do, you're liable to take a fall. Second is to be relaxed. A relaxed driver is more capable of observing the surroundings and responding to them than is one who hunches rigidly over the wheel and whose very stiffness inhibits the ability to observe and react to the surroundings and any situations that might occur. And, both exhibit the need for an upright, seated posture that facilitates movement that originates from the core of the body.

I once thought I could find poetry anywhere. Eventually, I learned I was wrong, but even so, it's in a lot of places. Same with Tai Chi. Like outside in my driveway.

Complex patterns of "correspondences" reaches its highest pitch of perfection in the East, where cosmic allegories (such as the Wheel of Transformations, the Yang–Yin disk, the Shri-Yantra, etc.) provide a most intense, graphic expression of these notions of contradiction and synthesis. The basic elements of such antithesis are the positive principle (male, lucid, active), and, opposing it, the negative principle (female, obscure, passive); psychologically speaking, these correspond respectively to the conscious and unconscious components of the personality; and, from the point of view of Man's destiny, they correspond to involution and evolution. These symbolic figures therefore are not so much an expression of the duality of the forces involved, but rather of their complementary character within the binary system.

—J.E. Cirlot
A Dictionary of Symbols

Part IV

Natural Patterns

14. Mathematical and Mechanical Systems that Exhibit Tai Chi Behavior

I used the chapters of the preceding section to illustrate how one can find correspondences between Tai Chi and a number of apparently unrelated objects and processes. I'll continue in that same vein in this section to show how Tai Chi is rooted in physics and mechanics on both a physical level and an energetic one. It should come as no surprise that its physical and energetic movements can be observed within mathematical and mechanical systems. Undoubtedly, there are many such systems of which I am unaware, but I've found a number of them that illustrate my point and shed some light on Tai Chi.

Perhaps one of the easiest parallels to observe is alluded to in the statement from the Tai Chi Classics: "Seek the straight in the curved and the curved in the straight." This statement describes the idea that straight lines can drop into curves and that curves can throw off tangents. An excellent example can be seen in the action of the driving wheel of a railroad locomotive. Like tai chi, a driving wheel uses an offset of linear force in relation to an axis of rotation. (Figure 14.1) Normally, the wheel is spun using the linear force of the thrusting and counter-thrusting piston to create spin. But it also is possible to spin the wheel to drive the piston back and forth. The wheel's axis of rotation is like Central Equilibrium, and the piston is like an arm that is thrust forward or backward by the rotation of the wheel around its axis.

There are a number of other mechanical and mathematical systems that exhibit Tai Chi concepts, behavior, and dynamics. Please be aware that my descriptions of these systems are shallow. I am not a scientist, mathematician, or engineer, and the majority of the technical information on these systems comes straight from the *Wikipedia* entries on them—as do many of the illustrations. But I do know a little about Tai Chi and how particular types of movements can empower or be empowered by chi flow as well as by particular sorts of physical movements and impulses. What I'm getting at in the following examples is not a deep understanding of the systems, per se, but how these systems reflect and are reflected by Tai Chi principles and movements. These are admittedly "gee-whiz" sorts of essays, but I think that these systems help demonstrate how closely Tai Chi adheres to the mechanisms that underlie reality.

This is the power known to science as energy, to the Melanesians as *mana*, to the Sioux Indians as *wakonda*, the Hindus as *shakti*, and the Christians as the power of God. Its manifestation in the psyche is termed, by the psychoanalysts, libido, and its manifestation in the cosmos is the structure and flux of the universe itself.

—Joseph Campbell
Hero with a Thousand Faces

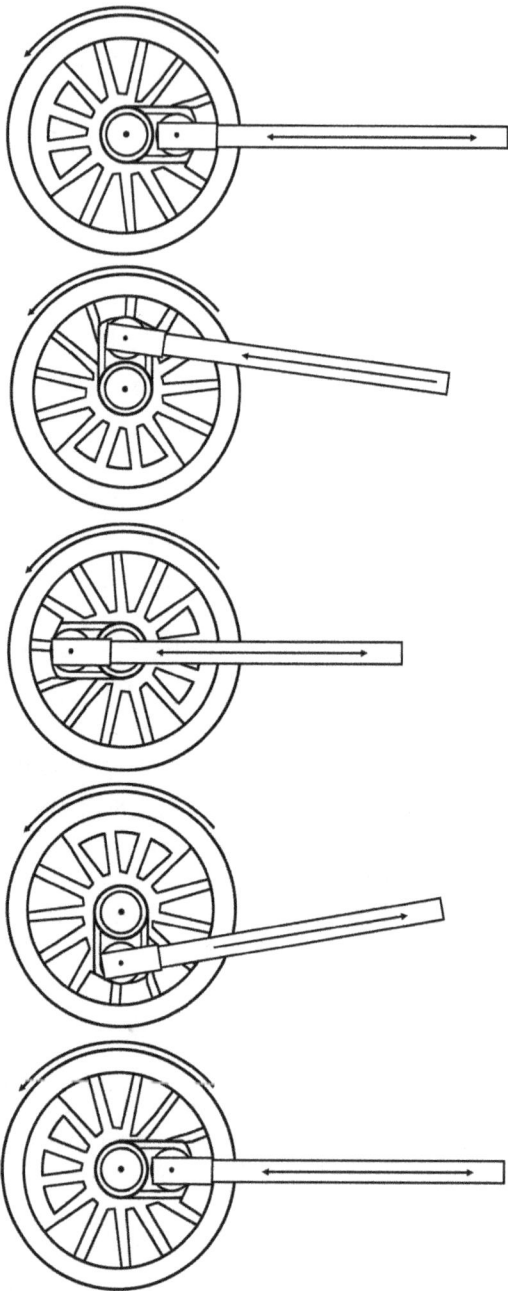

Figure 14.1 The driving wheel of a locomotive utilizes an offset of linear force in relation to an axis to create propulsion. It also illustrates the way the body converts linear force into circular movement and vice versa.

15. Lemniscate

We'll start with the lemniscate and its variants. (Figure 15.1) The term comes from Latin and means "decorated with ribbons." In algebraic geometry, a lemniscate is any of several figure-eight or ∞-shaped curves. Lemniscate are considered to be cross-sections of a torus. (Figure 15.2) If a torus is bisected by a plane parallel to the axis of the torus, the result in most cases is two circles or ovals. (Figure 15.3) However, when the plane is tangent to the inner surface of a torus—like slicing a donut right at the inner edge of its hole—the cross-section takes on a figure-eight shape, or, a lemniscate.[1] The illustration of the Cassini Oval clearly demonstrates the torus shape in profile. (Figure 15.4)

The variations between the several types of lemniscate are of interest primarily to mathematicians and scientists, but the Tai Chi Chuanist will readily recognize the basic shape as being the essence of the doubled tai chi symbol. (Figure 15.5) I've written extensively about how force and energy cycle through the doubled taijitu in my book, *Circling the Square: Observations on the Dynamics of Tai Chi Chuan*, and elsewhere in *Taijitu Magazine*, so I won't reiterate all that here except to say that Tai Chi Chuan is so named because its movements, both physical and energetic, rely for their power on follow-

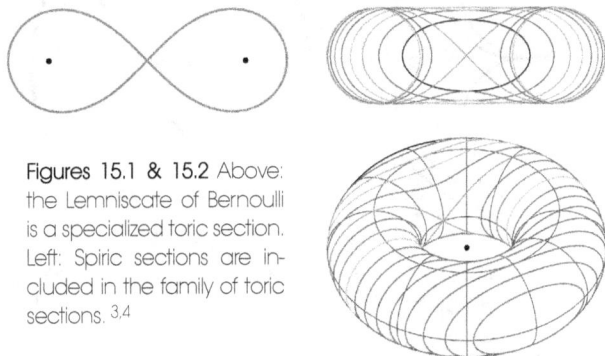

Figures 15.1 & 15.2 Above: the Lemniscate of Bernoulli is a specialized toric section. Left: Spiric sections are included in the family of toric sections. [3,4]

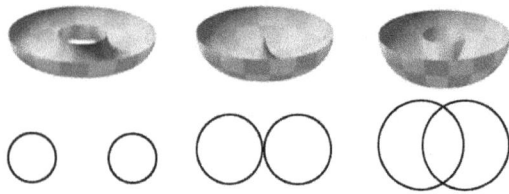

Figure 15.3 Bottom halves and cross-sections of the three classes of torus. From left: ring torus, horn torus, and spindle torus.[5]

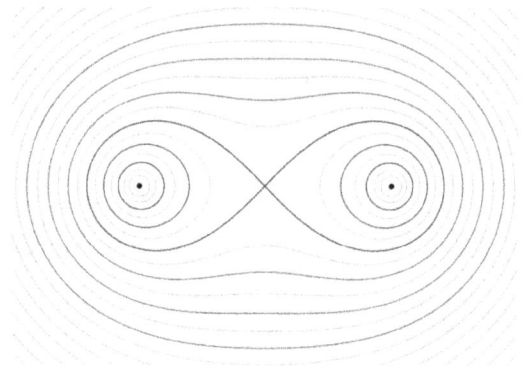

Figure 15.4 Some Cassini ovals.[7]

ing the path—or some portion of it—of the curves—particularly the figure-eight in the middle—found in the doubled taijitu.

This fact becomes even more interesting when one further considers the torus itself, which is the structure of which lemniscate are subsets. "A torus is a surface of revolution generated by revolving a circle in three-dimensional space about an axis coplanar with the circle."[2] Looking at a picture, it's easy to conceive of a torus as a static donut shape, but while inner tubes, bagels, O-rings, and even apples and red blood corpuscles are toroidal shapes, they are not true tori, but are solid torus shapes. A solid torus is formed by rotating a disc around an axis and is the torus plus the volume of matter inside the torus. A true torus is formed by rotating a ring around the axis, and the resulting form is empty yet energetic. (Figure 15.6)

A true torus is anything but static. It is in constant motion, but that motion isn't a simple rotation in one direction, like the rolling of a wheel. Instead, the

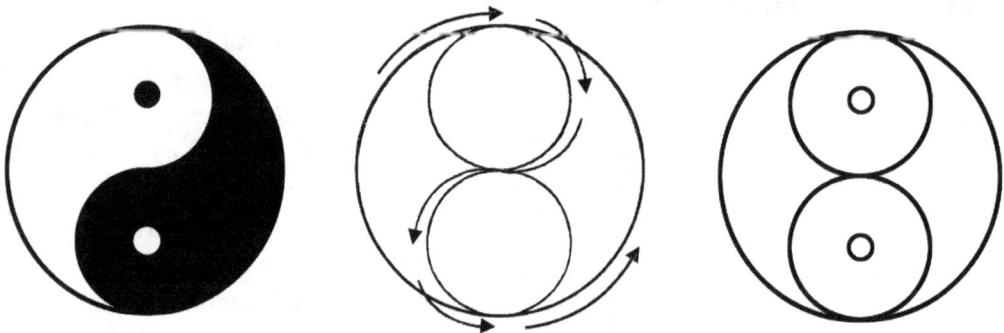

Figure 15.5 The taijitu as usually depicted, indicates clockwise rotation. By threading the energy through the center, the rotation can be reversed without pausing the energy's momentum. This action, done repeatedly, creates a figure eight at the heart of the taijitu.

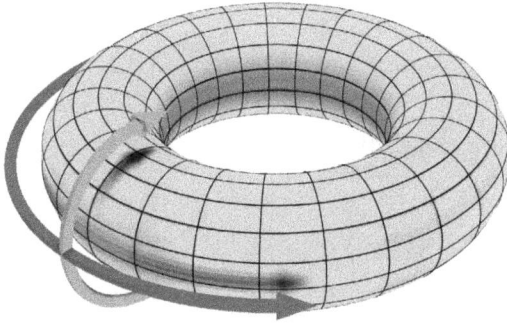

Figure 15.6 A torus is the product of two circles rotating at right angles to one another.[6]

torus is in constant movement in two dimensions, which anchors it within three dimensions. Two examples of energy tori are the magnetic fields that surround magnets, the Earth, and many other celestial bodies. The biofield that surrounds the human body also is a torus.

The implications for Tai Chi are that the movements of the art do not simply orbit through the figure-eight in one direction or the other, but that the entire figure-eight also constantly and simultaneously spins toward and away from the onlooker. These complex yet unified movements allow a person who has developed the skill of sensing and riding these currents the ability to rotate, spin, or otherwise avoid incoming force along any curve or tangent and then to cause the force to come back upon itself or to become enveloped in the practitioner's energy.

The animation of a punctured torus is a case in point. (Figure 15.7) Consider the torus to be the tai chi exponent's field and the point of puncture to be the opponent's incoming energy. As soon as the incoming energy penetrates the torus field, the exponent melts away then rolls and folds back from the point of entry. At all times, the torus exhibits emptiness to the force, yet the torus remains a torus. Another interesting case is how a torus in four dimensions—the three spatial ones over a span of time—almost magically turns force that is moving in one direction into force that moves in a tangential direction. (Figure 15.8)

The interesting thing about a torus is that, like ovoids, it seems to have multiple sides—front and back, at least—but at all times, it actually presents only one face to the outside. In essence, it can eternally cycle around itself without stopping or reaching an end. One example of this is the Möbius Strip (Figure 15.9), which is a toroidal section that has only one side.[10] If an ant were to crawl steadily along a Möbius Strip, it would make two revolutions and end up just where it started. In tai chi, some hand movements mimic the twist of the Möbius Strip or some portion of it. (You can create a Möbius Strip by cutting a strip of paper, giving the strip one twist, and taping the ends together. Presto! You have a created a two-dimensional structure that has finite width and infinite length within three-dimensional reality.)

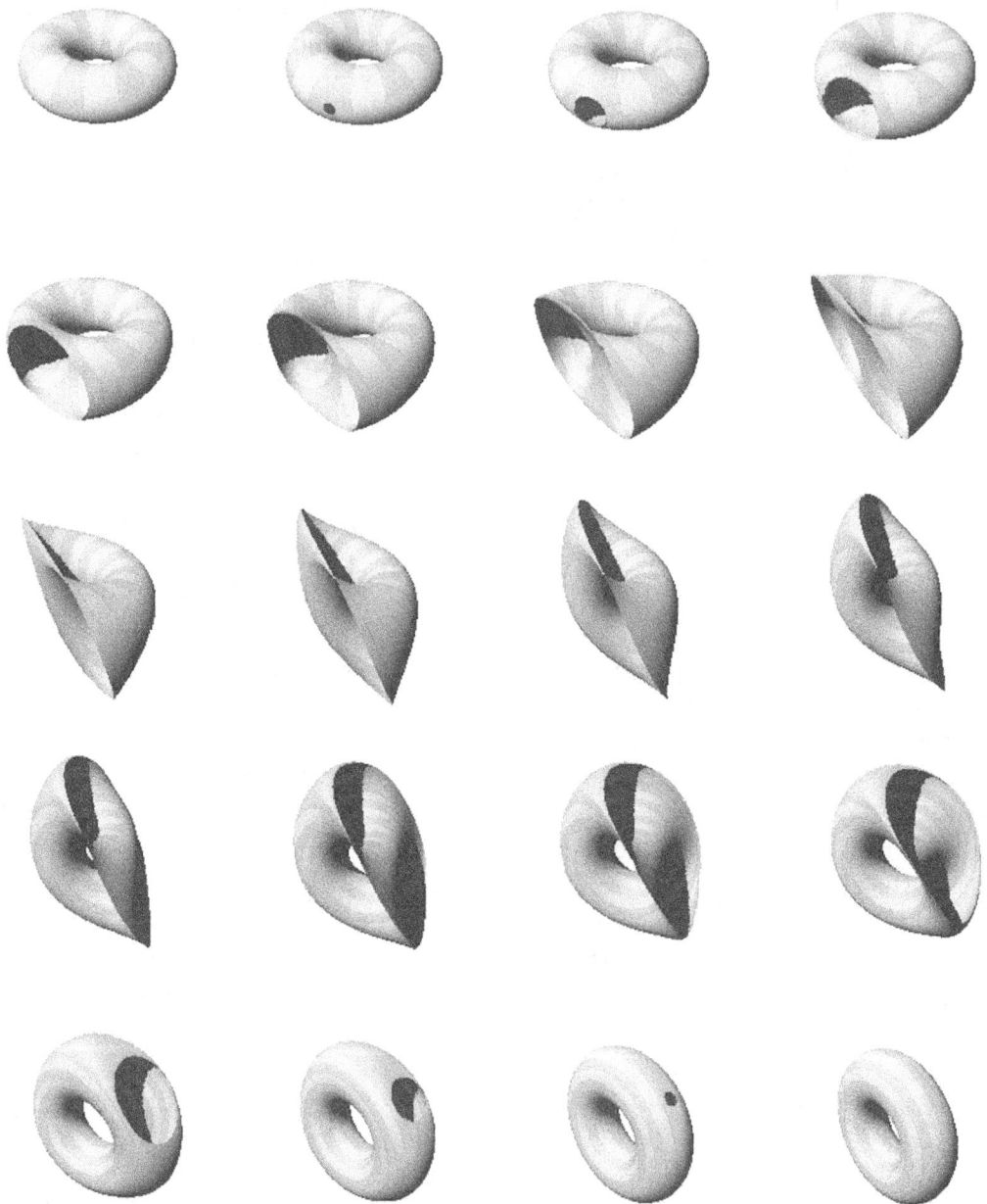

Figure 15.7 A punctured torus in motion. Interestingly, as the puncture in the wall expands and folds back, it becomes the next donut hole, opening into emptiness.[8]

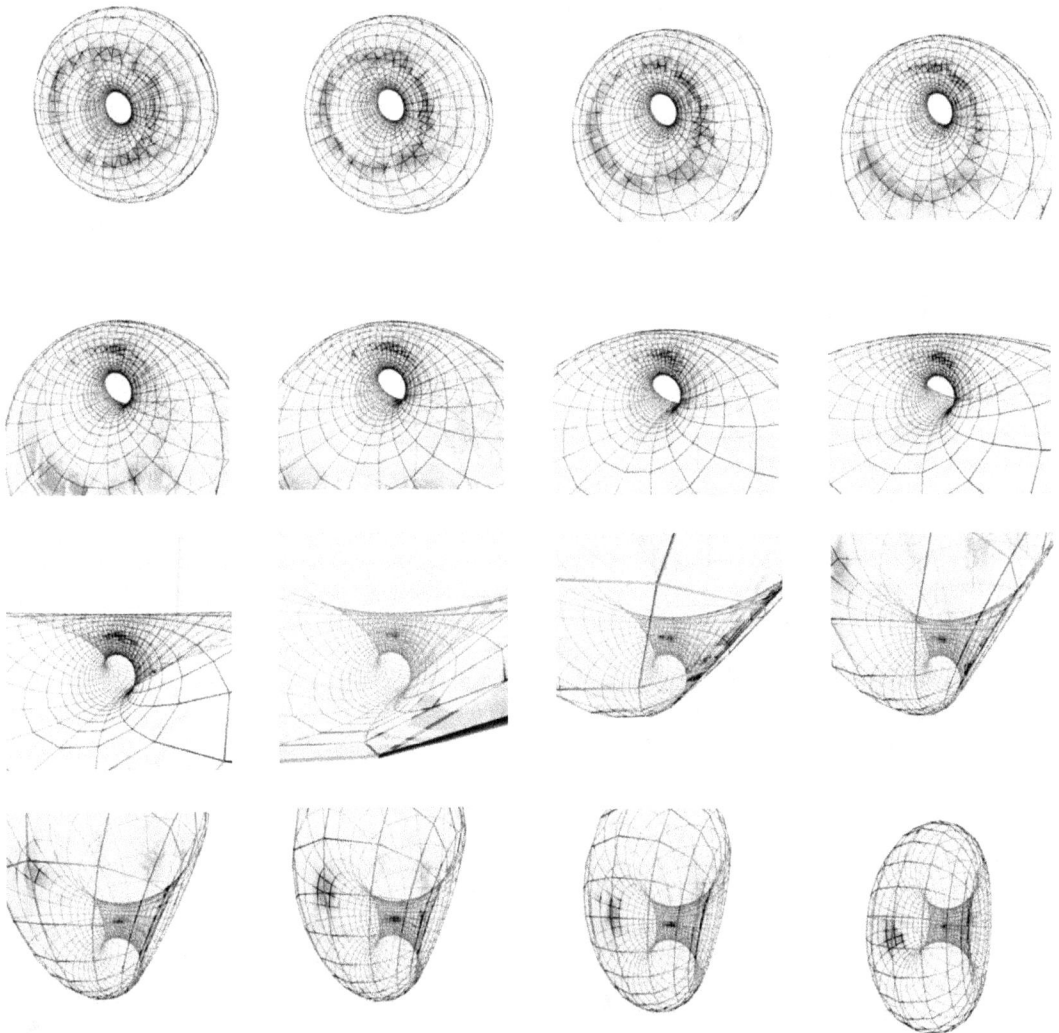

Figure 15.8 A stereographic projection of a Clifford Torus in four dimensions performing a simple rotation through the x-z plane.[9]

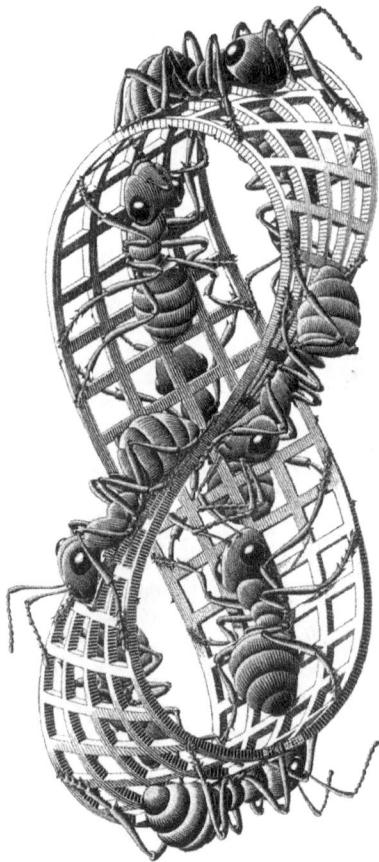

Figure 15.9 A Möbius Strip is a section of a torus in which the infinite nature of the shape is easily seen. This famous one is by M.C. Escher.[11]

Circumference

A symbol of adequate limitation, of the manifest world, of the precise and regular, as well as of the inner unity of all matter and all universal harmony, as understood by the alchemists. Enclosing beings, objects, or figures within a circumference has a double meaning: from within, it implies limitation and definition; from without, it is seen to represent the defence of the physical and psychic contents themselves against the perils of the soul threatened from without, these dangers being, in a way, tantamount to chaos, but more particularly, to limitation and disintegration.

—J.E. Cirlot
A Dictionary of Symbols

16. Spiral

Spiral. The very word elicits the movement of the line that creates the figure from a specific central point to an arbitrary periphery—arbitrary because, of course, a spiral theoretically spirals outward forever. Spirals abound in nature, and mathematicians have identified a great number of types. All of them illustrate not only the functionality of Tai Chi but also its universal beauty. We'll start with the simple basic spiral known as the Archimedean Spiral or arithmetic spiral. (Figure 16.1) This is a spiral whose successive turns are equidistant from each other in a simple arithmetic progression: 1, 2, 3, 4, etc. In other words, each turn is the same distance from the turns next to it, no matter how large the spiral grows.

Archimedean Spirals can be found in watch balance springs, the grooves of early gramophone records, and products bought in rolls, such as wrapping paper, tape, and vinyl flooring. It also can be used, interestingly enough, in one method of mathematically squaring a circle, and we all know that one of Tai Chi's precepts is to find the straight in the curved and the curved in the straight. Or to turn Tai Chi's four principal energies—the Cardinal Energies of Wardoff, Roll-

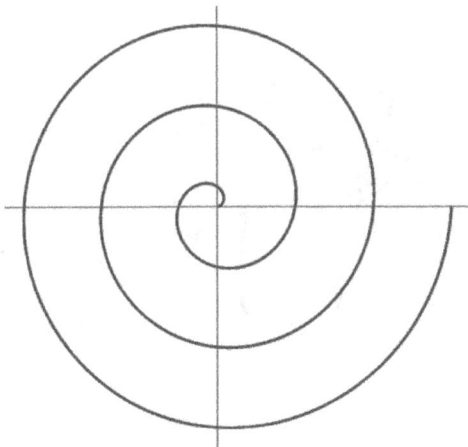

Figure 16.1 Three 360° turnings of one arm of an Archimedean Spiral.[4]

back, Press, and Push—into an infinite variety of circular and spiraling movements.

A more technical reading of the definition of an Archimedean Spiral is interesting from a Tai Chi standpoint: Such a spiral corresponds "to the locations over time of a point moving away from a fixed point with a constant speed along a line which rotates with constant angular velocity."[1] Think of performing a simple Rollback without any sort of flinging or pulling. The Tai Chi exponent is the fixed point, while the opponent is the one rolling away from the fixed point with a constant speed and constant angular velocity.

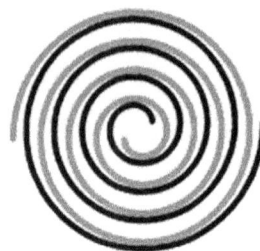

Figure 16.2 Mechanism of a scroll compressor.[5]

One interesting application of the Archimedean Spiral can be found in the mechanism of a scroll compressor (Figure 16.2), which is used to compress gases and liquids. In the illustration, the gray spiral is stationary because of the device's function, but it wouldn't be similarly constrained inside a dynamic system such as the human body. Imagine these two spirals as an energy structure within the torso or the individual limbs, and that you're looking lengthwise at it, with both spirals revolving: the black spiraling inward

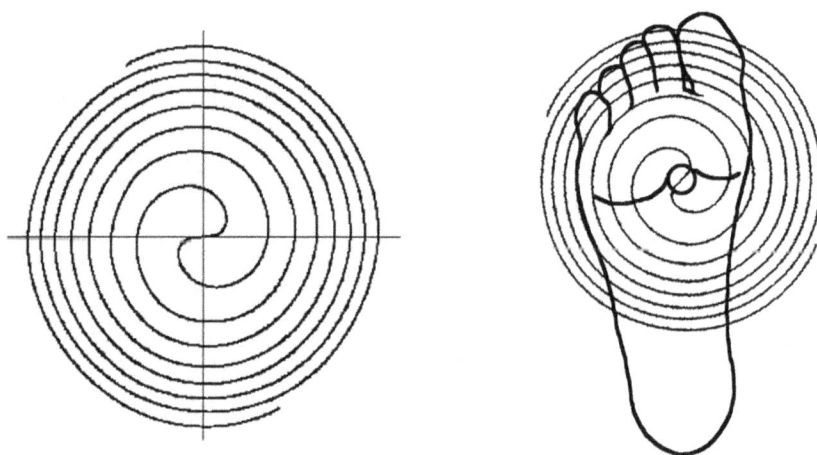

Figure 16.3 Fermat's Spiral demonstrates how energy spiraling inward can change direction without pause or loss of momentum. Tai Chi uses this spiral to channel force and energy down the leg and into the sole of the foot, where they change direction at the Bubbling Well, located in the hollow of the foot just behind the ball and front pads, before spiraling back up the leg. The spiral can twist in either direction, down or up, depending on the purpose of the movement.[6]

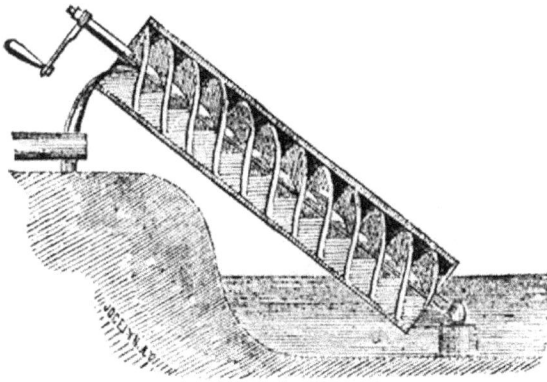

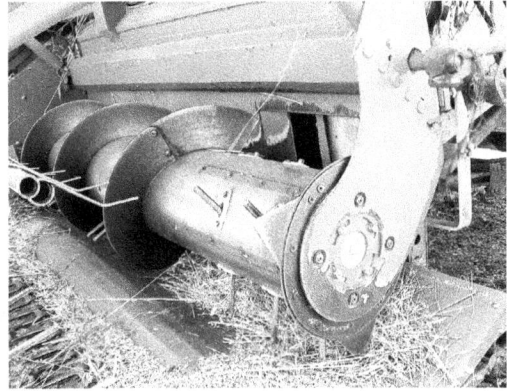

Figure 16.4 Archimedes' Screw is a device that can transport matter from one level to another. Originally it was a hand-operated device for lifting water in the ages before mechanical pumps, left. A combine harvester, right, is a modern use of Archimedes' Screw. [7,8]

and the gray outward. This is very similar to the way that you can spiral chi energy downward or outward then back in the opposite direction, compressing it in the process, much in the same way that the scroll compressor squeezes gases or liquids. Chi, after all, is a fluid energy.

The energy's change in direction at the central point—at the Bubbling Well of the foot in Tai Chi—is well-illustrated by a type of Archimedean Spiral called Fermat's Spiral. (Figure 16.3) It's easy to see in the diagram how energy spiraling inward can smoothly change direction without stopping so that it can spiral outward without losing momentum. You also can see that the curve where the change in direction takes place is like the S-curve running through the taijitu.

Before we leave the well-regulated world of the Archimedean Spiral, let's look at one more practical application of this structure: the Archimedes Screw. (Figure 16.4) This is a device for lifting—pumping—water commonly attributed to Archimedes but that probably is older by several hundred years. More recently, the device has found uses in other types of machinery, such as combine harvesters. (Figure 16.4) The interesting point for Tai Chi Chuanists is the way that screwing or spiraling energy can propel an object along a line perpendicular to the circular action. (Figure 16.5)

Archimedean Spirals are nice and regular thanks to their simple arithmetic progression, but another class of spiral exhibits a logarithmic progression, unwinding with turns that are wider and wider at a regular mathematical rate, such as 2, 4, 8, 16, etc., or 3, 9, 27, 81, etc. (Figure 16.6) Such spirals open up faster than they turn. One Archimedean Spiral will look like all other Archimedean Spirals, but the mathematical variety of logarithmic spirals means that such spi-

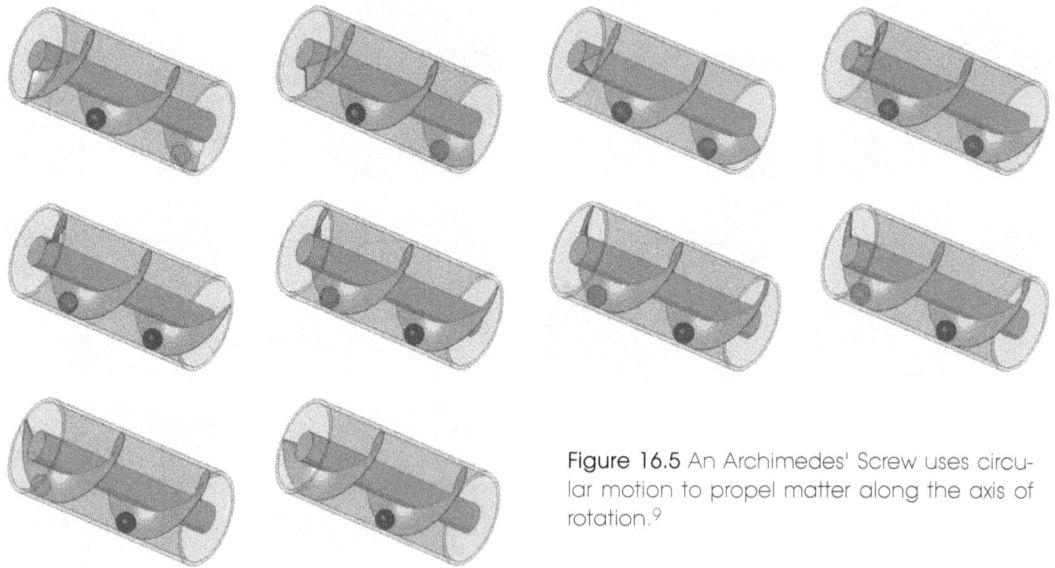

Figure 16.5 An Archimedes' Screw uses circular motion to propel matter along the axis of rotation.[9]

rals can take a large number of exact forms, though they might have a class-based similarity in appearance.

Logarithmic spirals are widely found in nature: in sea shells, hurricanes, flower petals, spiral galaxies, and much more. It's even found in the Mandelbrot Set, which mathematically describes the boundary between order and chaos. (Figure 16.7) This also is the boundary that lies between the Tai Chi exponent (order) and incoming energy (chaos) that is manipulated by the Tai Chi exponent by exploiting these spirals.

Logarithmic spirals are frequently employed in engineering. One example is the Euler Spiral (Figure 16.8), which finds application in railroad engineering to create ideal transitions from straight runs of track as they lead into curves, and vice versa. Appropriate angles of curvature help transit the forward momentum of the train smoothly into and through the curving track so that the train experiences minimal tilt. This is yet another example of finding the straight in the curved and the curved in the straight.

One group of logarithmic spirals called the Cote's Spiral can either spiral outward or inward. (Figure 16.9) These actions of loga-

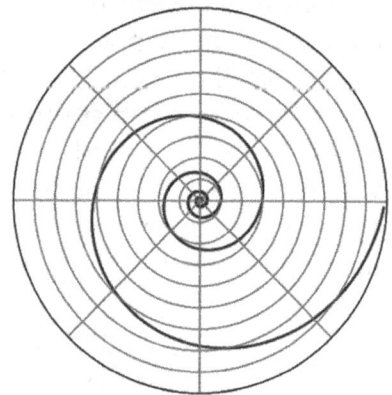

Figure 16.6 A logarithmic spiral opens faster than it turns.[10]

rithmic spirals are employed by the Tai Chi Chuanist when Rollback is combined with an outward flinging or an inward pulling.

One very special logarithmic spiral is produced from a mathematical concept that is called the "Golden Ratio." Mathematically, the Golden Ratio occurs when the ratio of two quantities is the same as the ratio of their sum to the larger of the two quantities. In other words, where *a* is the larger quantity, there is a golden ratio if *a+b* is to *a* as *a* is to *b*.[2] Mathematicians since Euclid have studied the properties of the Golden Ratio. In 1202, the Italian mathematician Fibonacci (Leonardo Pisano Bigollo) published a sequence of numbers—called the Fibonacci Sequence—that approximates the Golden Ratio, and this sequence has found application in computer algorithms, graphs, and other scientific and mathematical techniques. The mathematics of the Fi-

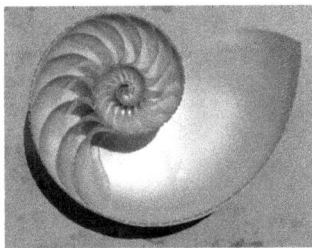

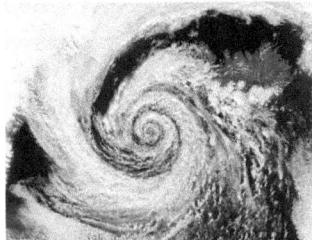

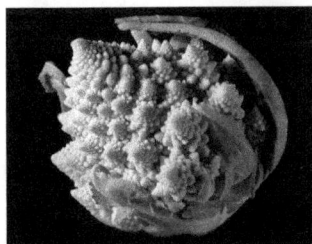

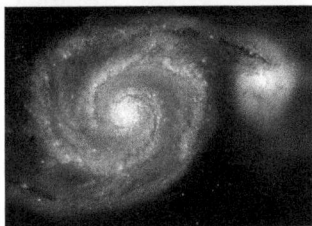

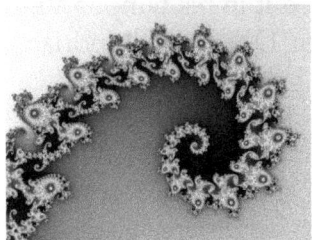

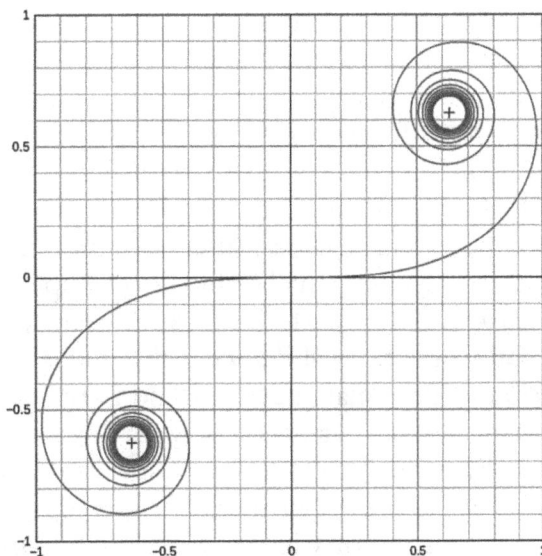

Figure 16.7 Logarithmic spirals abound in nature, including the Mandelbrot Set (bottom), which mathematically describes the boundary between order and chaos.[11]

Figure 16.8 The Euler Spiral finds application in railroad engineering to create ideal transitions from straight runs of track as they lead into curves.[12]

bonacci sequence can be graphically depicted in the design of the "Golden Spiral." (Figure 16.10)

Indeed, the Golden Ratio is called the "divine proportion" because it is ubiquitous in natural physical structures, such as the branching of trees, the arrangement of leaves on a stem, the fruit sprouts of a pineapple, the flowering of an artichoke, the uncurling of a fern, the arrangement of a pine cone, the veins of leaves, the spiral form of some mollusk shells, and many others.

Adolf Zeising, whose main interests were mathematics and philosophy, found the Golden Ratio expressed in the skeletons of animals and the branching of their veins and nerves, the proportions of chemical compounds, and the geometry of crystals. The Golden Ratio's ubiquitous presence throughout nature prompted him to see it as a universal law of natural structure. In 1854, Zeising wrote that this universal law "contained the ground-principle of all formative striving for beauty and completeness in the realms of both nature and art, and which permeates, as a paramount spiritual ideal, all structures, forms and proportions, whether cosmic or individual, organic or inorganic, acoustic or optical; which finds its fullest realization, however, in the human form."[3]

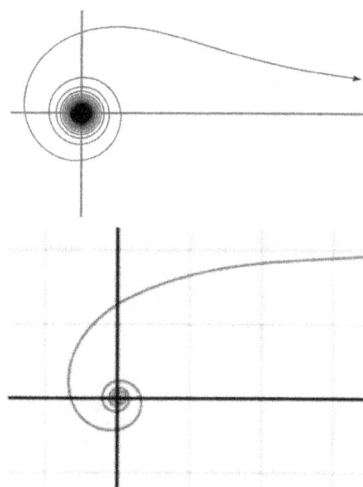

Figure 16.9 Two examples of Cote's Spiral: The Litus, top, spirals outward, while the hyperbolic spiral, above, arcs inward.[13,14]

Naturally, artists as well as scientists and mathematicians have been fascinated with the Golden Ratio. Leonardo Da Vinci roughly displayed it in his famous Vitruvian Man, and it has been used more recently by Salvador Dali, Piet Mondrian, and others. One extremely obvious example is Johannes Vermeer's *Girl with the Pearl Earring*. (Figure 16.11) The Argentinean sculptor, Pablo Tosto, has listed more than 350 works by well-known artists whose canvasses feature the Golden Ratio or a close approximation. It is found in the architecture of the Great Mosque of Kairouan, and the famous Swiss architect Le Corbusier extensively used the Golden Ratio in his designs. It also is present in the proportions of Medieval manuscripts, and even in music. Musicologist Roy Howat has observed that the formal boundaries of Claude Debussy's *La Mer* correspond exactly to the Golden Ratio, although it is disputed whether this was deliberate or not.

For Tai Chi enthusiasts, the Golden Ratio should have its own special meaning, particularly when it is converted, using the Fibonacci Sequence or other

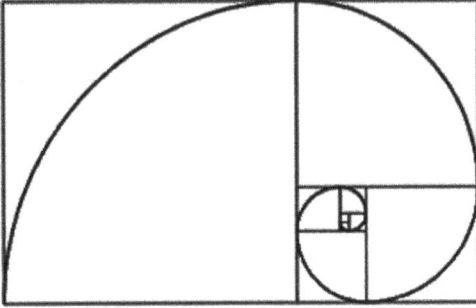

Figure 16.10 The Golden Spiral, a foundation of order and beauty in nature, resembles a single taijitu fish.

techniques, into the previously mentioned visual representation called the Golden Spiral. The Golden Spiral is a logarithmic spiral that gets wider by a factor of the Golden Ratio for every quarter turn it makes. One look at this spiral, and you will instantly see what I mean. A single spiral is similar to one tai chi symbol fish, and when the spiral is doubled, it forms an approximation of the entire tai chi symbol—or, rather, the taijitu approximates a doubled golden spiral. (Figure 16.12)

Figure 16.13 illustrates how the taijitu and the Golden Spiral can work together to draw incoming energy into a vortex and then expel it through an unwinding of the vortex, similar to Fermat's Spiral, mentioned above. It

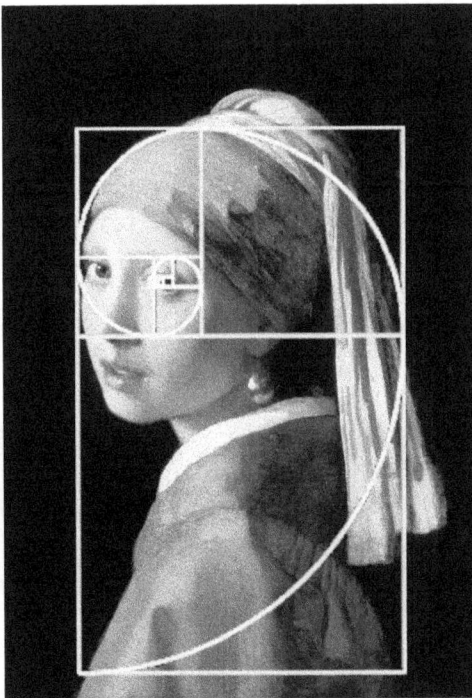

Figure 16.11 Johannes Vermeer's *Girl with the Pearl Earring* illustrates one way that artists have incorporated the Golden Spiral into their work.

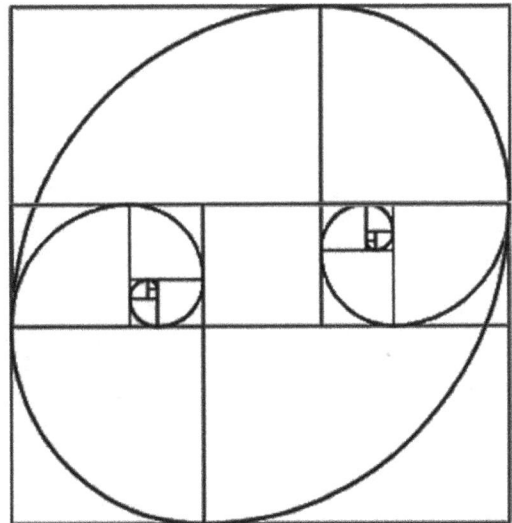

Figure 16.12 When the Golden Spiral is doubled,, it creates a figure resembling the tai chi symbol.

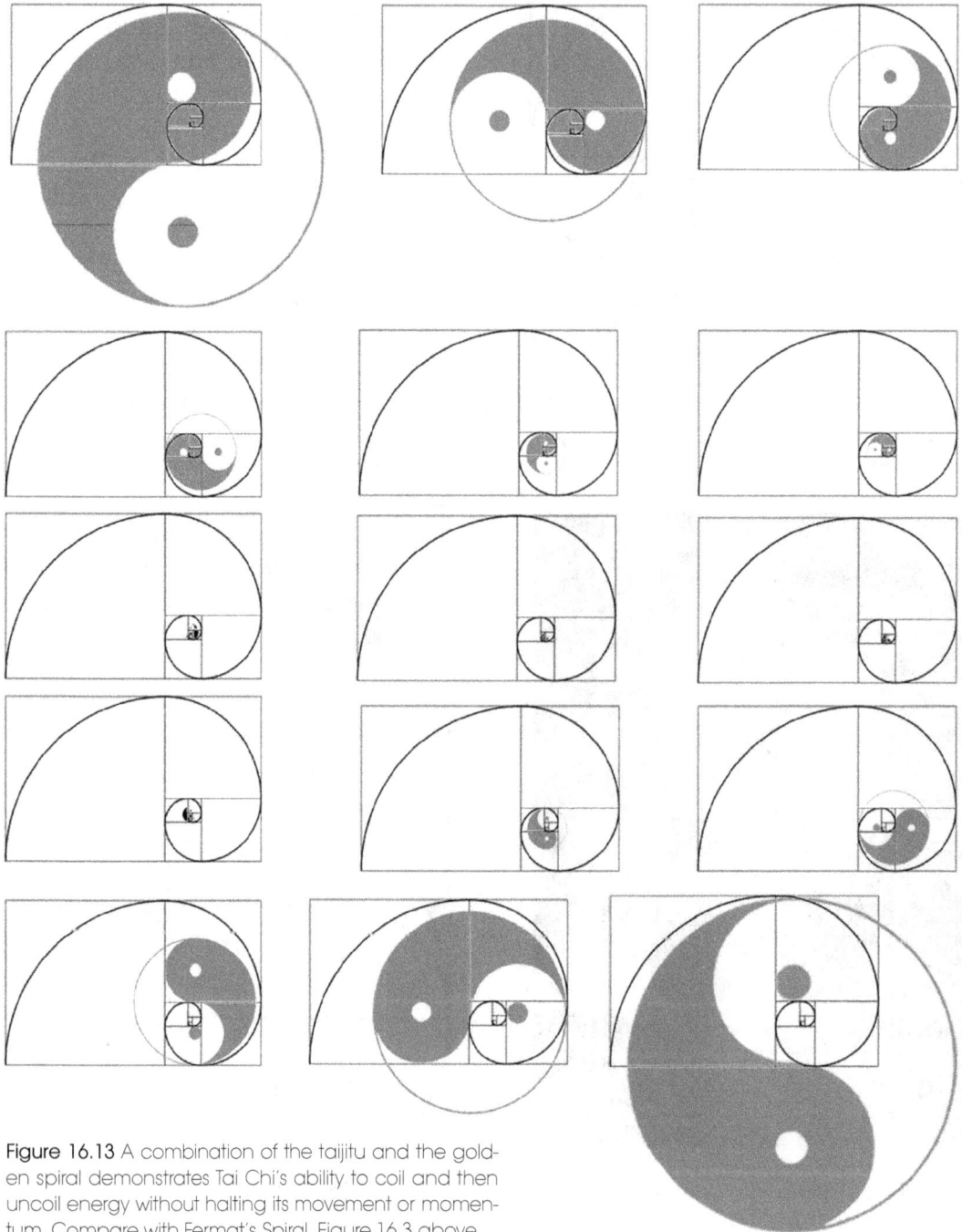

Figure 16.13 A combination of the taijitu and the golden spiral demonstrates Tai Chi's ability to coil and then uncoil energy without halting its movement or momentum. Compare with Fermat's Spiral, Figure 16.3 above.

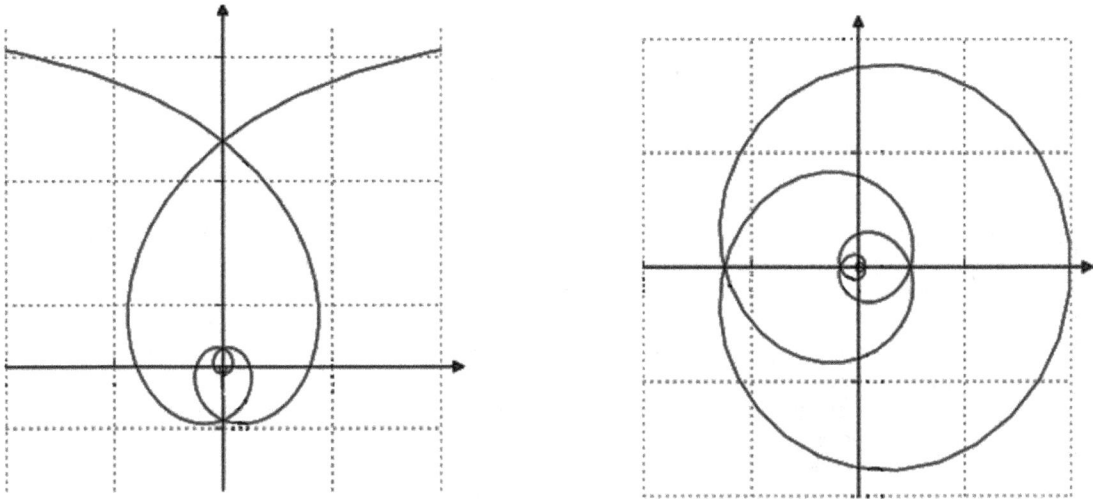

Figure 16.14 Two Poinsot's Spirals, one open, one closed. Many Tai Chi movements follow the path of this spiral, or some portion of it.[15]

also demonstrates the fact that Tai Chi, like the taijitu and the Golden Ratio, is fractal: No matter what its scale, it always takes the same form and operates on the same principles.

Before we leave spirals, let's look at one more: Poinsot's Spiral. (Figure 16.14) This is an altogether more complex logarithmic spiral that spirals back upon itself. Interestingly, the way that chi energy spirals through the major portion of Grasping Bird's Tail in Northern Wu Style, if viewed from above, almost perfectly mimics the entire Poinsot's Spiral. And many other Tai Chi movements utilize various portions of it.

Tai Chi movements often are described as circular, but in reality the descriptor should be "curvilinear" or "spiraling," for the art takes advantage of movements that expand or contract along curving lines, leading to spirals or other non-ending curvilinear structures, such as parabolas and hyperbolas. Over time and with practice, the spirals that begin by being large expressions of physical movement contract, becoming small spirals that exist almost exclusively inside the body, spiraling downward and upward through the torso and legs and outward and inward along the arms.

Spiral

A schematic image of the evolution of the universe. It is also a classical form symbolizing the orbit of the moon, and a symbol for growth, related to the Golden Number, arising (so Housay maintains) out of the concept of the rotation of the earth. In the Egyptian system of hieroglyphs the spiral—corresponding to the Hebrew *vau*—denotes cosmic forms in motion, or the relationship between unity and multiplicity. Of especial importance in relation to the spiral are bonds and serpents. The spiral is essentially macrocosmic. The above ideas have been expressed in mythic form as follows: "From out of the unfathomable deeps there arose a circle shaped in spirals.... Coiled up within the spirals, lies a snake, a symbol of wisdom and eternity." Now, the spiral can be found in three main forms: expanding (as in nebulae), contracting (like a whirlwind or whirlpool) or ossified (like a snail's shell). In the first case it is an active sun-symbol, in the second and third cases it is a negative moon-symbol. Nevertheless, most theorists, including Eliade, are agreed that the symbolism of the spiral is fairly complex and of doubtful origin. Its relationship with lunar animals and with water has been provisionally admitted. Going right back to the most ancient traditions, we find the distinction being made between the creative spiral (rising in a clockwise direction, and attributed to Pallas Athene) and the destructive spiral like a whirlwind (which twirls round to the left, and is an attribute of Poseidon). As we have seen, the spiral (like the snake or serpent and the Kundalini force of Tantrist doctrine) can also represent the potential centre as the example of the spider's web. Be that as it may, the spiral is certainly one of the essential motifs of the symbolism of ornamental art all over the world, either in the simple form of a curve curling up from a given point, or in the shape of scrolls or sigmas, etc. Parkin observes in his *Prehistoric Art* that "no ornamental motif seems to have been more attractive than the spiral. Ortiz suggest that, from a semantic point of view, the spiral is an emblem of atmospheric phenomena and of the hurricane in particular; but the fact is that the hurricane in its turn is a symbol of secession from the creative (as well as destructive) functions of the universe, that is, of the suspension of the provisional but pacific order of the universe. He also points to the connection between breathing and the creative breath of life. He goes on to suggest that the volute in ancient cultures was a spiral form symbolizing the breath and the spirit. It is for this reason that the Egyptian god Thoth is represented with a large spiral on his head. Finally, by virtue of its significance in connexion with creation, with movement and progressive development, the spiral is an attribute of power, found in the sceptre of the Egyptian pharaoh, in the *lituus* of Roman augurs, and in the present day walking stick. In addition to the above, it is also possible that the spiral may symbolize the relationship between the circle and the centre. For the spiral is associated with the idea of the dance, and especially with primitive dances of healing and incantation, when the pattern of movement develops as a spiral curve. Such spiral movements (closely related to the pattern of the mandala and the spiral form that appears so frequently in art from the Mesolithic Age onwards—particularly in France, Ireland and England) may be regarded as figures intended to induce a state of ecstasy and to enable man to escape from the material world and enter the beyond, through the "hole" symbolized by the mystic Centre.

—J.E. Cirlot
A Dictionary of Symbols

17. Curve

Curves can be considered to be sections of circles/spheres, tori, and spirals. Tai Chi exponents are acutely aware of the importance of curves in a basic sense, but some curves demonstrate that the form of curves isn't always simple. We saw above how the taijitu, and particularly its central curvilinear line, forms or is a section of a spiral. Most of us probably think of the figure-eight produced by a reverse doubling of the taijitu as being flat, but that isn't necessarily the case within three-dimensional reality. Instead, the taijitu should be visualized as a three-dimensional torus, with an infinity of possible curves and spirals rotating around and through it. When moving in three dimensions, one can spiral in one direction then change the angle of the motion to continue spiraling without a break in another direction that is not only tangential, but perpendicular to the first.

This fact is important in Tai Chi as a way to smoothly lead the direction of incoming force into another path. Generally, the Tai Chi exponent is thought of as being a sphere that simultaneously backs away from and turns away from an incoming force. This can happen on a simple physical level, but one extremely interesting mathematical curve shows how incoming force can be enveloped by an energetic sphere in preparation for manipulation. This is Viviani's Curve, which is the result of a cylinder impinging itself upon a sphere.

Not all such impingements will produce the same result. If the cylinder completely penetrates the center of the sphere, the intersections will be two circles, and if it does not fully enter the sphere, the intersection will be something like a bite taken from an apple. But if the cylinder is allowed to penetrate the sphere only as far as its back edge, the result is Viviani's Curve, a figure-eight that also is called the Lemniscate of Gerono that completely wraps the cylinder and can exert spiraling influence on the cylinder from any angle and toward any angle. (Figure 17.1)

If you map the figure of the Lemniscate of Bernoulli onto Viviani's Curve, the former seems to warp inward at the ends, making the structure more akin to one of the two leather skins that wrap a baseball, unfolded, than to a flat depiction. Thus, the eyes of Bernoulli's figure—of the taijitu fishes—are where the cylinder's axis touch the surface of the sphere depicted in Viviani's Curve. This means that the energy cycling through the loops of Viviani's Curve completely encases the cylinder's one-dimensional axis with three-dimensional energy.

The Watt's Curve, named for the inventor James Watt,

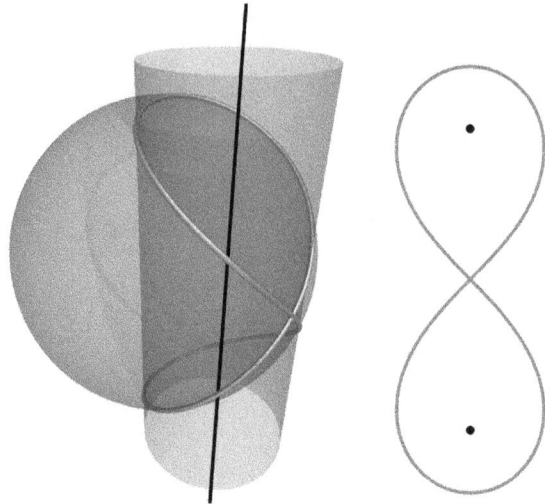

Figure 17.1 Viviani's Curve (left) results from a sphere wrapping a cylinder exactly to its edge. The figure suggests a three-dimensionality to the taijitu that is not immediately obvious in the flat symbol. When considered as the central figure-eight of the taijitu, the Lemniscate of Bernoulli (right) maps in very interesting ways onto Viviani's Curve, suggesting a three-dimensionality to the taijitu that isn't immediately obvious from the two-dimensional taijitu.[1,2]

is yet another complex curve that demonstrates Tai Chi principles of movement. (Figure 17.2) Thankfully we have animations to show how energy can be cycled through the complex yet basic taijitu circles and figure-eights to propel energy in certain manners because I don't think I could possibly describe the movements with words. Several ways of looking at these systems apply to Tai Chi. For example, when looking at the three moving points, consider the central one to be Central Equilibrium and the other two to be the hands at the ends of the arms. It can be seen how relatively small yet stable and centered movements can propel much larger swings of energy as one leads the energy through the different curves and junctions, particularly the figure eights.

James Watt gave us another Tai Chi example in a simple mechanism called the Watt's Linkage. (Figure 17.3) This mechanism shows how external force acting on an object with a Tai Chi center can be diverted by moving through the curve

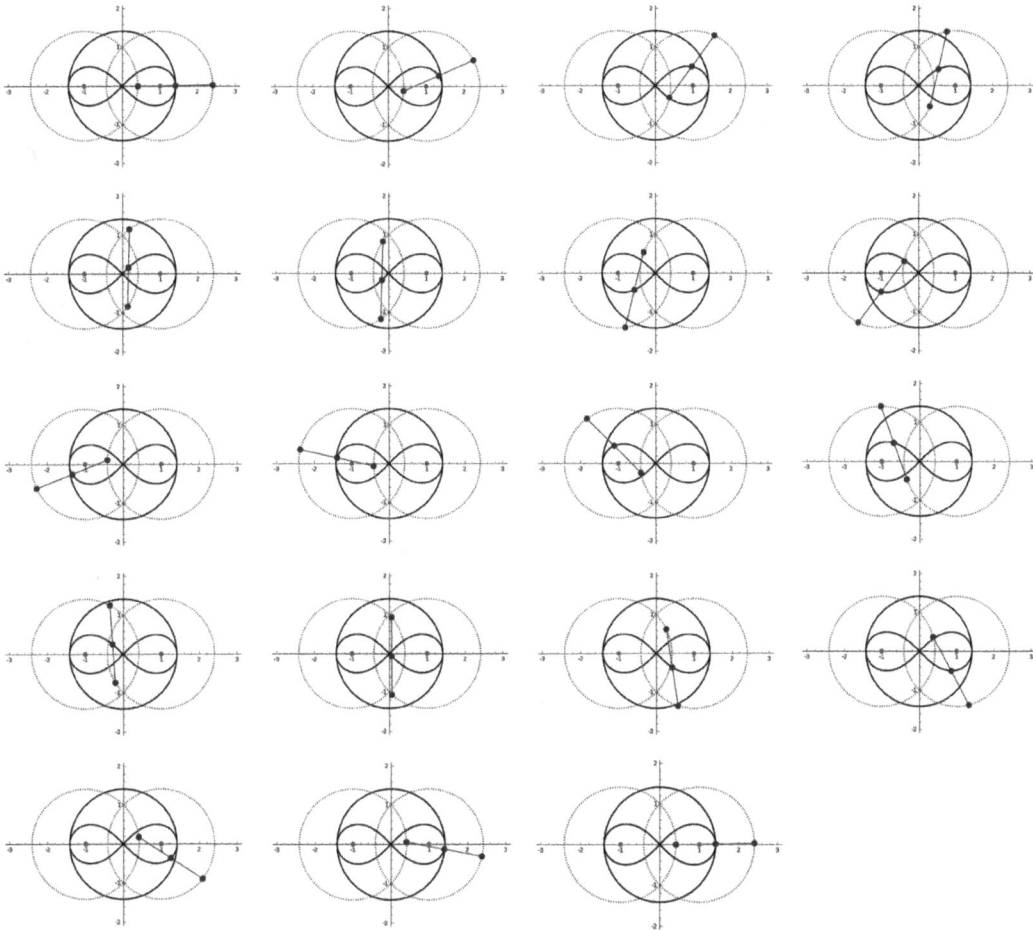

Figure 17.2 One of several forms of Watt's Curve. In the animation, pay attention to the movement of the armature consisting of a dark line with three dots (at the center and on both ends) as it cycles through the figure. The animation shows only one half of the complete cycle.[3]

in the middle of the taijitu. Conversely, it shows how the taijitu S-curve can instigate angular momentum. Both are additional examples of finding the straight in the curved and the curved in the straight.

Still another example of the straight and curved is the Trammel of Archimedes, which, when made from wood and sold in roadside joints, is sometimes called the Kentucky Do-Nothing. (Figure 17.4) It derives this latter name by being a device that is interesting but that has no apparent real function, though

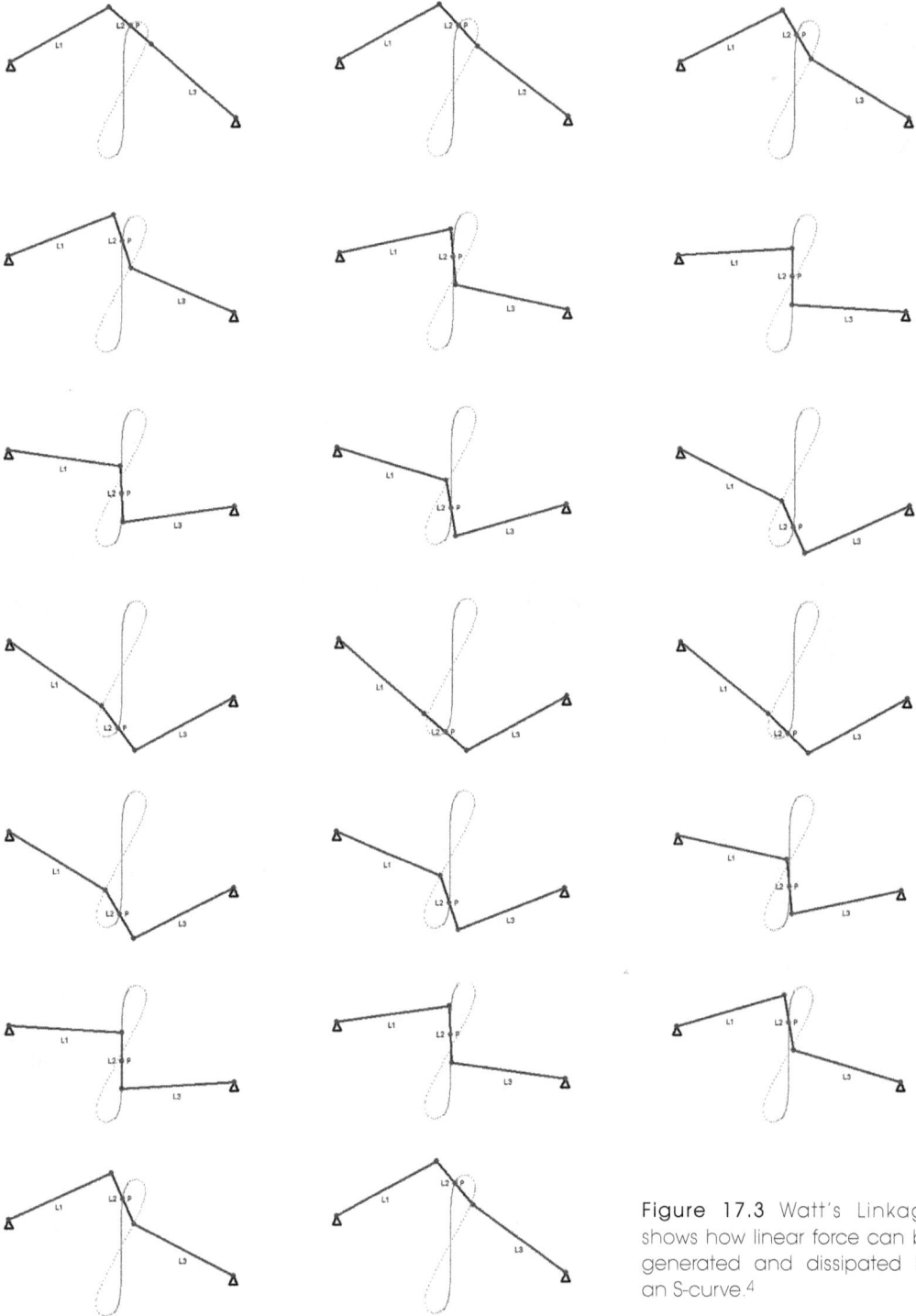

Figure 17.3 Watt's Linkage shows how linear force can be generated and dissipated by an S-curve.[4]

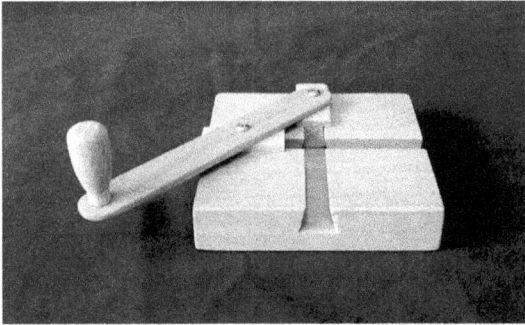

Figure 17.4 A nice example of a Kentucky Do-Nothing.[5]

the Trammel of Archimedes is used as a method to draw or cut ellipses. (Figure 17.5) But from a Tai Chi perspective, it perfectly illustrates how two linked linear forces can produce not only an ellipsis but can be used to fling an object to some distance or pull it inward.

This is another device that you can look at in several ways, say with the center of the cross in the middle as Central Equilibrium, the two sliders as the hands, and the black square as the external force or opponent; or the black square can be the Tai Chi exponent, the farther slider the opponent, and the near slider the pivot point between them. As with all of these systems, you can find your own parallels.

Tai Chi teachers emphasize many different aspects of the art, such as relaxation, continuity, chi development, martial applications, and so forth, but throughout all these aspects runs one unifying concept: naturalness. This naturalness seems to come from the movements, but in truth, the power of the movements stem directly from their perfect adherence to nature, from its most superficial aspects to its deepest reaches.

Curl

In the Egyptian system of hieroglyphics, the loop is a determinative sign defining the ideas of either binding or unbinding, depending upon the position of the loose ends. It corresponds to the general symbolism of bonds and knots.

—J.E. Cirlot
A Dictionary of Symbols

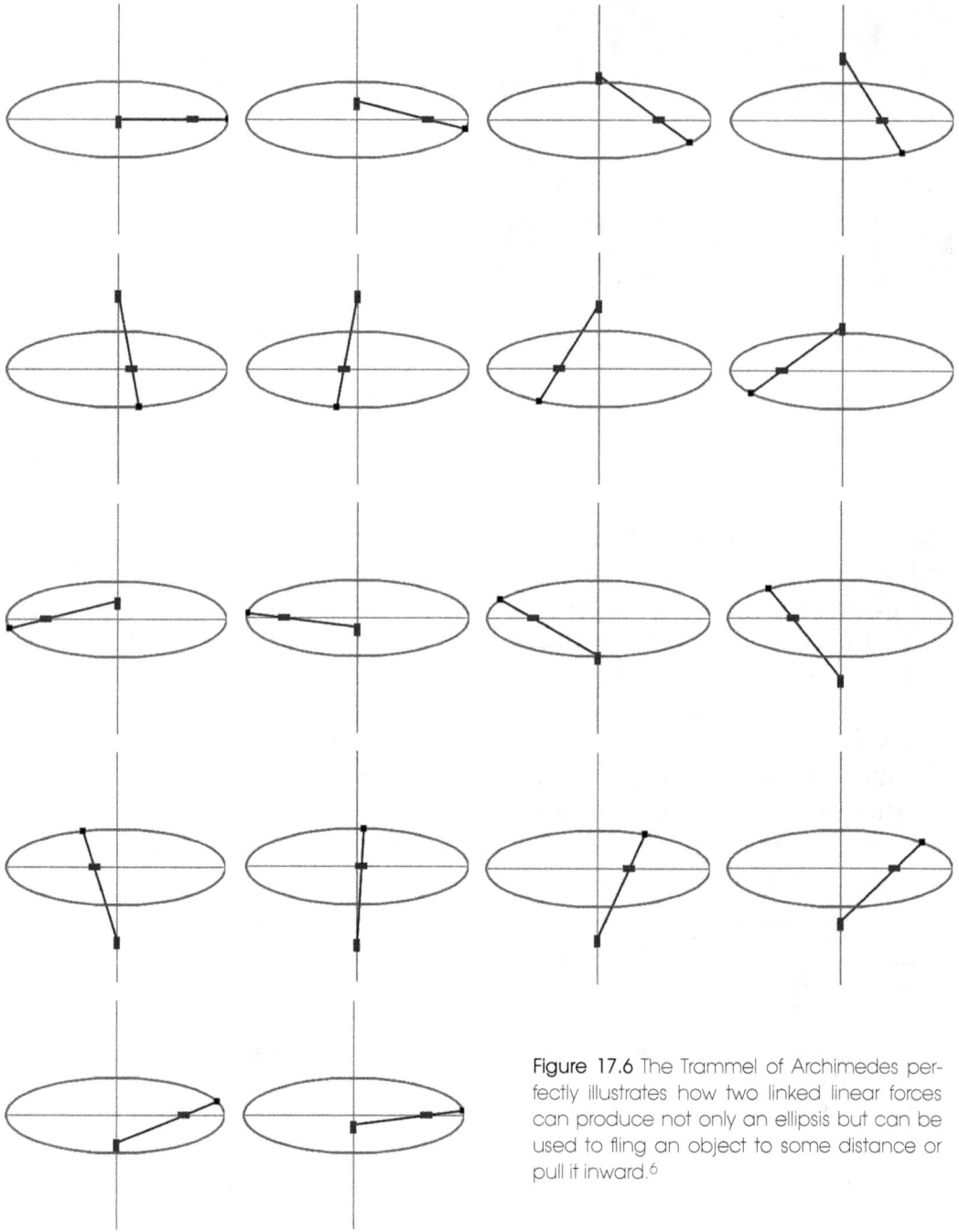

Figure 17.6 The Trammel of Archimedes perfectly illustrates how two linked linear forces can produce not only an ellipsis but can be used to fling an object to some distance or pull it inward.[6]

18. Mutual Interaction

The first episode of the BBC documentary, *Edge of the Universe*, is about the search for extraterrestrial planets. Even the closest stars that contain planetary systems are so far from Earth that it is impossible to spot their planets directly. Not only are the planets of other solar systems too small to see, even for the most powerful telescopes, such objects are lost in the glare of their home suns.

But those suns hold the key to spotting their planets. Astronomers knew that if gas giants are orbiting a star, their gravitational pulls on their sun would cause the star to appear to wobble back and forth. Our gas giants—Jupiter and Saturn, primarily—do that to our sun, it's just that it takes decades of observation to detect even the slightest relative movement due to the extreme lengths of these planets' orbital periods. Eventually, though, astronomers began to spot such stars and, from the periodicity of their wobbles, could determine the approximate number, sizes, orbital distances, and orbital speeds of the gas giant or large terrestrial-type planets involved. The *Kepler* spacecraft, a space observatory launched in 2009, could detect much smaller planets, and to date, more than 4,000 exoplanets have been found by Kepler and other means, with thousands of candidates waiting in the wings for confirmation. Nearly 700 of those already confirmed are Earth-size. Not long ago, astronomers announced the discovery of an astounding seven terrestrial-type planets in a single system: Trappist-1.

The Tai Chi point in all of this is the wobbling dance of a star and its planets. The wobbles of stars with multiple planets, such as our sun, can be quite complex, but not so with the first exoplanet ever confirmed, which is a huge gas giant orbiting alone and quite close to and quite rapidly around the star 51 Pegasi. The BBC program had a nice animation of the interaction between the two bodies, and it is almost exactly like the movement embodied in the Trammel of Archimedes, discussed in the previous chapter. In a very real sense, a single planet in such a situation doesn't just orbit the star; the planet and the star each orbit around a fixed point located along the direct line of gravitational force between the two objects. This fixed point is located, of course, much closer to the star than to the planet, despite this particular planet's considerable bulk and nearness to 51 Pegasi.

In essence, this is very similar to the interactive "dance" of a Tai Chi exponent dealing with incoming energy, even if that energy isn't as neatly regular as forces acting on a planet constantly revolving in a nearly fixed orbit around a star. As an opponent launches the energy of an attack, which can come from a variety of angles and at different speeds, the exponent sinks, turns, and then performs one of the various actions that can follow to best deal with the incoming energy. In the case of a solar system like 51 Pegasi, both bodies might actually constantly rotate around one another, but the dynamics, from a Tai Chi perspective, are a little different.

From this perspective, the sun, having a stronger gravitational pull (chi) constantly rotates away from the mutual centerline gravitational pull (line of attack) between it and the planet (opponent), and the planet is flung to the side. But of course, the chi plus rotational ability of the Tai Chi exponent does not include the powerfully and mutually attractive force of gravity that exists between celestial bodies and which is constant and intractable, so the sun cannot actually fling away a planet that is in a regular orbit. But it does fling it—precisely enough to perfectly counteract the pull of gravity. This is what keeps the weaker-gravity planet in its orbit instead of falling inward. But the fact that the Tai Chi exponent isn't bounded or limited by gravity in the same way allows the exponent to deal in diverse ways with energy that is not in a neat orbital pattern by applying other actions in addition to flinging, such as striking, pushing, pulling, bouncing away, and so forth.

19. Doppler Style Tai Chi

Tai Chi Chuanists generally define their art within the microcosm of their body —or perhaps within a dynamic of their body's interaction with other bodies. But Tai Chi also closely adheres to broader natural laws. As I've shown elsewhere in this volume, it's not much of a stretch to find Tai Chi analogies within universal laws and phenomena. In this essay, we'll look for Tai Chi principles in what is commonly known as the red shift, although there also is a corresponding blue shift. Together, these two make up the yin and yang of the Doppler Effect.

The Doppler Effect is a phenomena of any energy that propagates through waveforms and produces a spectrum of intensities and frequencies, such as the electromagnetic spectrum or sound. The Doppler Effect is a product of the difference in the relative motion of the observer and the object that produces the waveform. Although, mysteriously, the speed of light is a constant no matter what an observer's velocity is, waves of light—and other associated energies and particles such as heat, radio waves, microwaves, and so forth—by their very nature, can be both stretched and compressed. They are compressed along the wave's front and stretched along the wave's wake. (Figure 19.1)

This elasticity of light waves becomes obvious in the character of light emanating from a star as it is measured by a distant observer. If the star is moving away from the observer, the light will be stretched toward the red and infra-red end of the spectrum, which has a longer wavelength. If the star is moving toward the observer, the light will be compressed toward the blue and ultraviolet end of the spectrum, which has a shorter wavelength. Cosmologists have used measurements of the red shifts of various galaxies to determine that most of them are moving away from the Milky Way, meaning that the universe is ex-

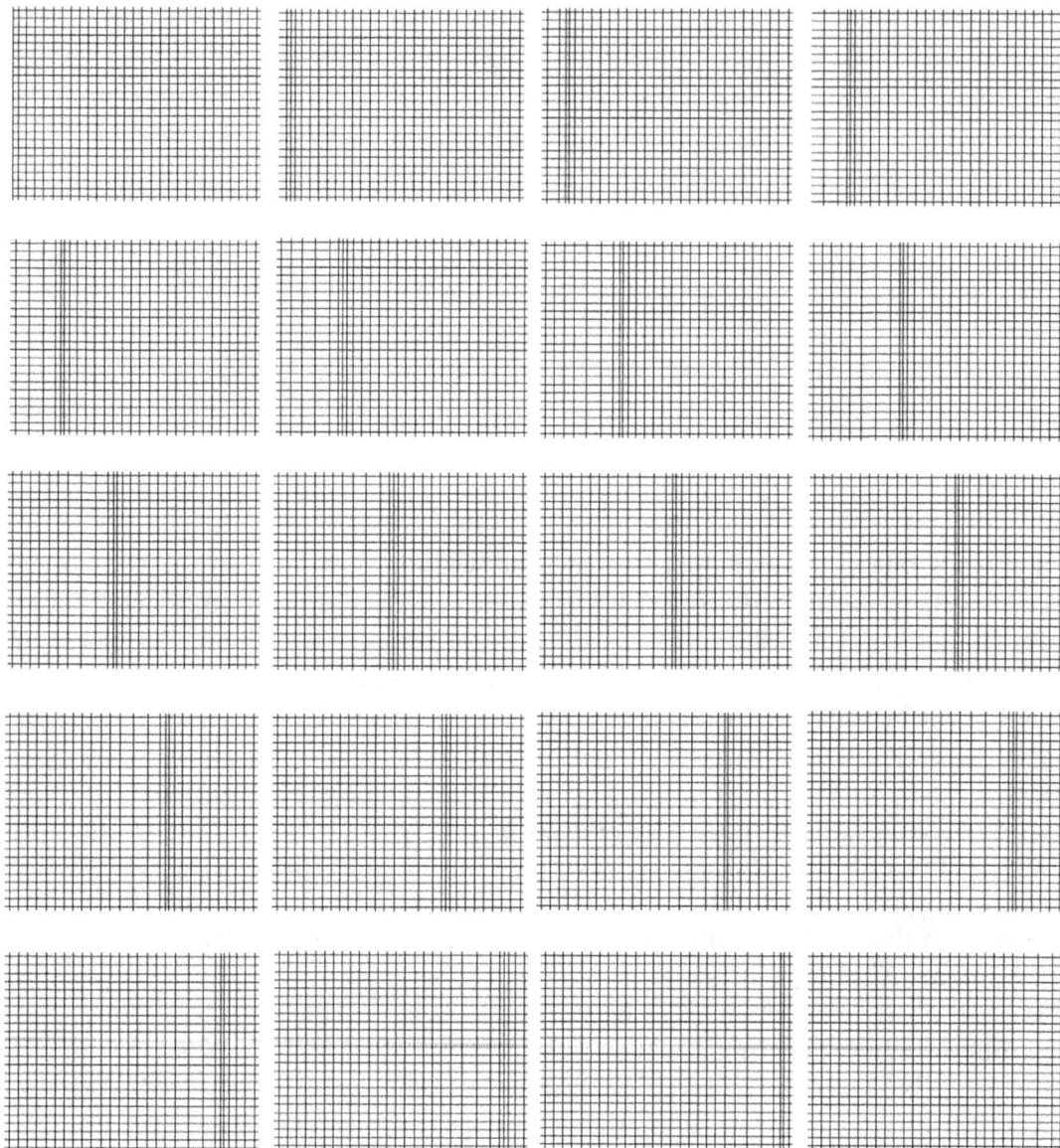

Figure 19.1 A unidirectional longitudinal wave (above) and an omnidirectional longitudinal wave (right). Both examples illustrate the compression and rarefaction of the medium through which the waves travel. Such waves also are called pressure waves because they produce increases and decreases in pressure.[1]

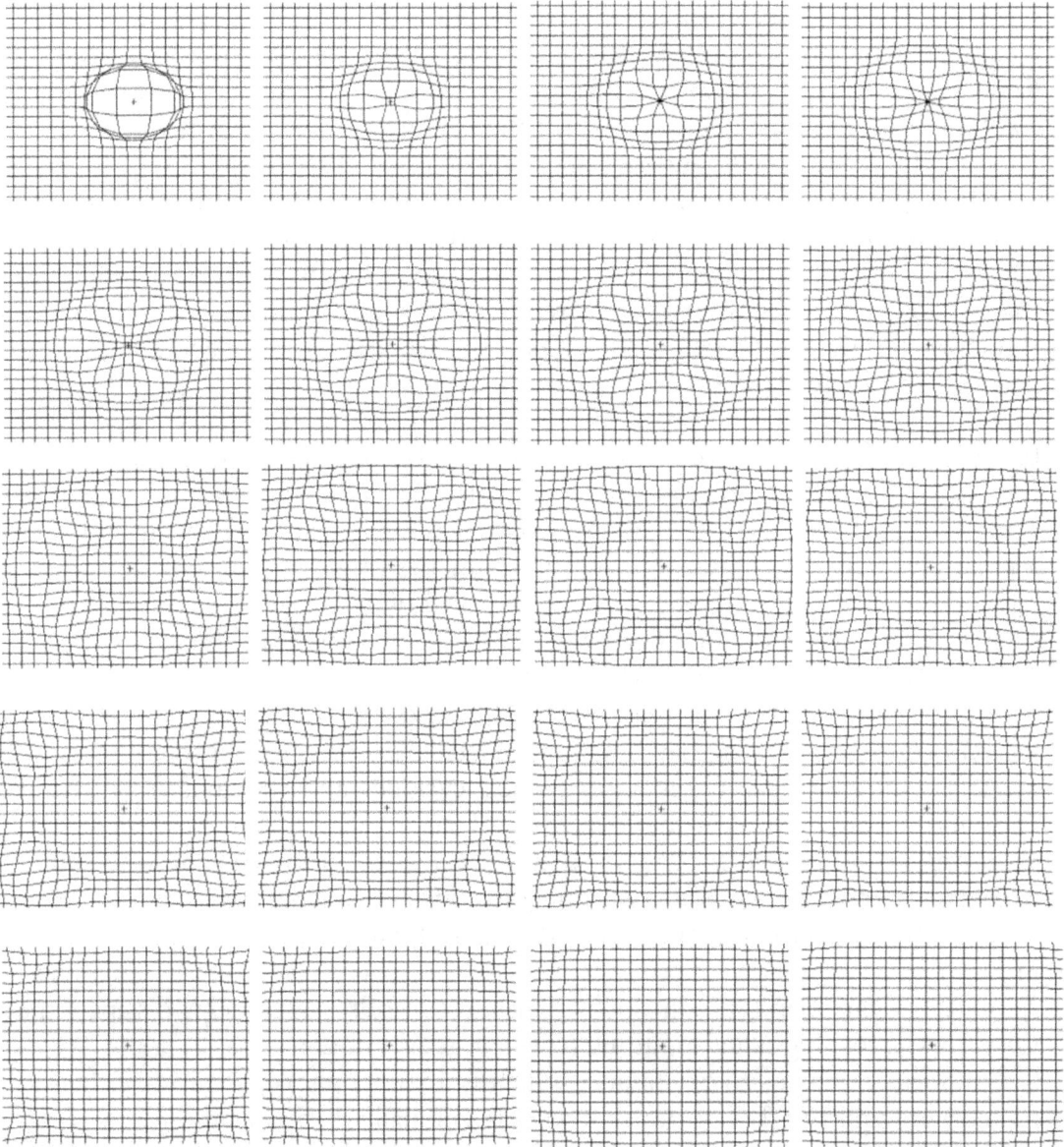

panding. However, there are a few galaxies that are moving toward us for one reason or another, and the light coming from these is compressed, shifting it toward the blue end of the spectrum.

The same phenomenon occurs with any energy that manifests in a waveform, such as sound, which produces the Doppler Effect in a way that is familiar to everybody. As a car approaches a listener, the sound of the engine rapidly rises in pitch, then, as the object passes and moves away from the listener, the engine sound suddenly drops in pitch. Both the increase and the decrease have nothing to do with the actual level of the sound—the volume—which has remained constant, but only with the degree to which the sound wave has been compressed as the car approaches the listener and then stretched as it moves away.

Of importance to Tai Chi Chuanists, the Doppler effect is an obvious expression of how a wave of energy can be either compressed or extended. And chi, being an electromagnetic energy that manifests as a waveform, is subject to the possibility of compression and stretching, too. Tai Chi folks call these manifestations fa jing, which can assume the role of yin or yang, depending on its particular mode of expression.

Yang fa jings are compressions of chi. In terms of elasticity, they either bounce or surge outward or squeeze inward. They usually have an element of focus—you're moving energy outward, with one degree or another of force, often homing in on a point, or squeezing something smaller or concentrating on a relatively small area of the body, even if for the briefest of instants. Interestingly, the compression of the surging chi of fa jing is often accomplished by sending a large wave down a narrowing channel, such as from the torso into an arm, all the way to the hand and fingertips.

This is tantamount to the magnified effect produced by a wave of water washing into an ever-narrowing bay. The low, coastal areas of the country Bangladesh are hit by an enormous number of tropical cyclones and tsunamis for just this reason. They are situated at the focal apex of any tropical storm or wave activity occurring in and around the Bay of Bengal, and woe to those people who find it necessary to inhabit such a region. They are constantly being washed out of their homes—and all too frequently, out of the ken of humankind. Ironically, though, in a sort of otherworldly response to the constant battering of all this yang energy, much of the inland terrain is slowly rising lowlands, which helps dissipate the yang force through gradual, uplifting (curving) redirection.

And this brings us to yin fa jing, which is a stretching of a chi wave. Just as the curving uplift of Bangladesh's lowlands gradually dissipates the force of cyclones and tsunamis, yin fa jing draws incoming energy into emptiness and diffusion. Or, alternately, instead of the explosion of yang fa jing, yin fa jing is an implosion that pulls or draws irresistibly toward its center. It is gravity, while yang fa jing is the opposite: momentum. And as we all know, stretching—or drawing a single object in opposite directions—produces a negative tension—in some instances an elastic storage of energy, as in a rubber band, in others a sucking sensation, as with a the undertow of a wave. Both are yin, but the former holds yang within the yin, while the latter is solely yin.

In a very real sense, the physical and energetic results of compression and expansion give substance to the statement from the Tai Chi Classics: When I attack, my opponent feels that he cannot retreat, and when he attacks, he feels that he cannot touch me. This is because the energy involved in compression and expansion flow with the movement and affect the opponent's own energy field, allowing the Tai Chi exponent a measure of control over it.

Furthermore, compression, being the yang version of elasticity, produces heat. Heat and repeated compression can temper materials like metals, refining them into something at once more useful and beautiful. Think of the Japanese sword maker, reheating, refolding, and hammering the metal of the blade as he forges an object of such incredible refinement that it can come alive in the hands of a master swordsman. Just the same, the heat and compressions of chi-building exercises on the body's psychophysical system produce refinements of the body, mind, internal energy, and spirit that lend positive qualities and greater control to one's own life. Remember: It's spiritual alchemy.

Diffusion, on the other hand, produces cold and distance and isolation. Cosmologists, observing the red shifts of distant galaxies, have determined that the universe is expanding at such a rate that it may actually be flying apart. Eventually, the only lights in the night sky will be those of the stars of the Milky Way and the handful of galaxies of our own galactic cluster—though possibly by that time, our own local cluster will have imploded into a single massive black hole.

And there you have it: the yang and yin of things on a cosmological level, with some stuff flying apart forever into infinity, and the same stuff simultaneously coalescing forever into singularities. In the meantime, for Tai Chi enthusiasts, we've seen a couple of more ways in which the principles of nature are mirrored in our art and practice. And I think we're safe enough for the moment, cosmologically speaking, so I'll hold off mourning the end of reality and keep on practicing.

> When the way comes to an end, then change—
> Having changed, you pass through.
>
> —I Ching

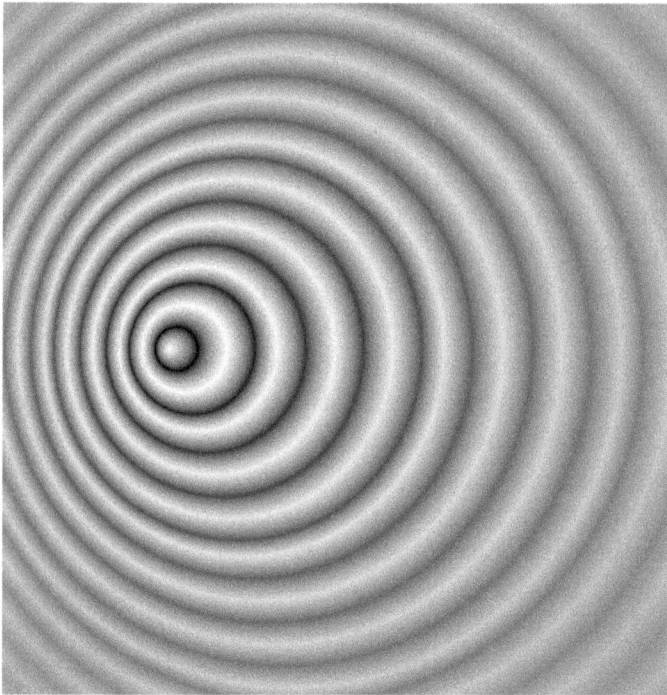

Left, a single circular compression wave. Below, two circular compression waves impinging on each other. The illustration clearly shows how such waves can amplify or cancel out each other.[2,3]

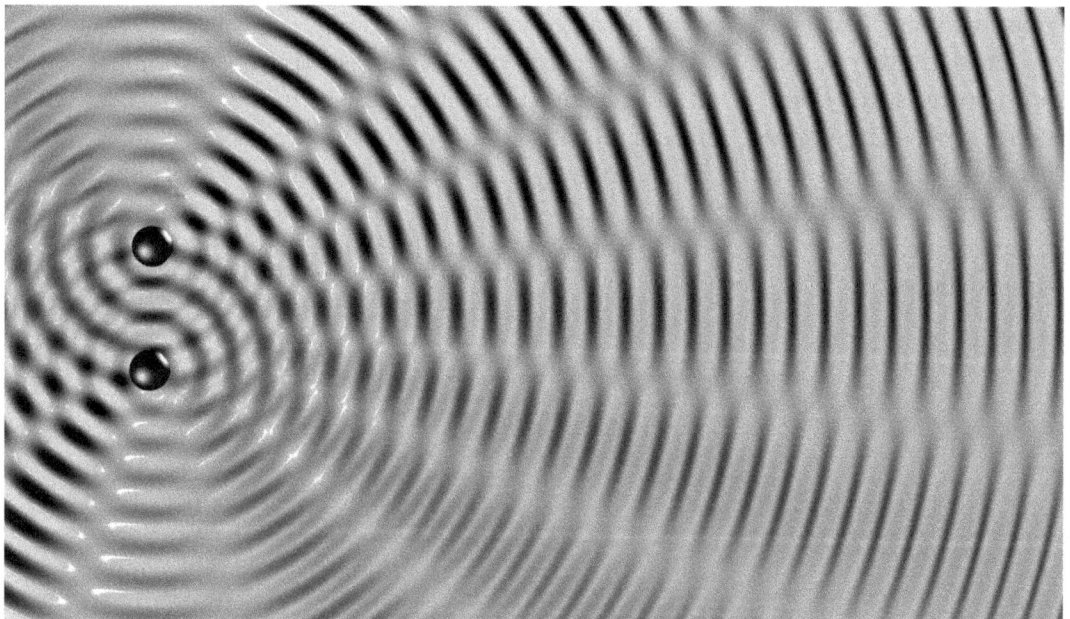

20. Tai Chi Under the Lens

Lenses aren't usually associated with Tai Chi Chuan. And why should they be? One is, most often, a specially shaped piece of glass or plastic, while the other is a complex physical movement discipline that functions in various ways. They aren't even apples and oranges, which are at least both fruit. They are so totally unrelated that they're more akin to something like apples and ball-point pens. But if you capitalize Apple, the computer can be considered a sophisticated version of mechanical instruments for writing and illustrating, of which ball-points also are examples. Perhaps, in many unexpected ways, lenses and Tai Chi, too, are more akin than is at first apparent.

Lenses aren't usually associated with food, either, but the name comes from the Latin name for lentil because a lens—at least in most magnifiers—is lentil-shaped. Nor are they usually thought of as toys. Lenses are serious business. They're in telescopes astronomers use to delve into the far reaches of the cosmos. They're in the microscopes modern medicine relies on to help identify disease. They're in the binoculars wielded by military commanders surveying their tactical options and in the Theodolites of surveyors who map our world. They're in the eyeglasses a great percentage of humankind depends on to see well. Naturally occurring lenses are in almost every eye.

I once read a news story about a fire at a liquor store that burned the place to the ground. The fire occurred during the middle of the day, and the proprietor saw nothing that could have caused the fire, which started at the front of the store, in the display area. Everything was normal one minute, and the next, the place was a raging inferno. Investigators determined that the culprit was the sun, whose rays coming through a window had been focused by a round bottle of clear liquor that acted like a lens. The focal point of all that burning energy was another bottle of alcohol, which, being highly flammable, went up like a Molotov cocktail. That set off the several hundred other Molotov cocktails lining the shelves. From there, the fire worked its way to the cases of Molotov cocktails in the storeroom, and then it was all over for that building. Lenses, it seems, really are serious business. They aren't toys.

But heck, almost as soon as I received my first dinky little hand-held telescope when I was about eight, I came into possession of another just like it. Almost instantly, one of them lay in pieces: hollow tubes, screw-on rings, O-ring clamps, and the precious guts comprising several lenses of different sizes. I valued these isolated lenses almost as much as I did the telescope that remained intact. The largest of them, I quickly observed, could start a fire when focusing sunlight. In that, I was simply replicating the experiments of my human forebears. The oldest known lens is the Nimrud Lens, which dates back to Assyria of the seventh century BCE and is now held in the British Museum. (Figure 20.1) It has been proposed that it and other ancient lens artifacts were used for much the same purposes that we use lenses today: to magnify things and start fires.

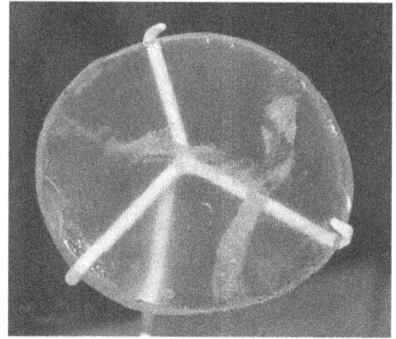

Figure 20.1 The Nimrud Lens, the oldest-known lens, dates to Assyria of the seventh century BCE. It is now held in the British Museum.[2]

Lenses are surprisingly complex business, too. There are six different types: biconvex, plano-convex, positive meniscus, negative meniscus, plano-concave, and biconcave. Convex is where the surface bulges out, and concave is where the surface curves inward, and the range is from lens that bulge out on both sides to ones that curve inward on both sides. (Figure 20.2)

But there is another property of lenses that is only partially tied to the lens's profile, and that is whether the lens is a positive/converging lens or a negative/diverging lens. The former focuses light—or other forms of energy in microwave lenses, electron lenses, or

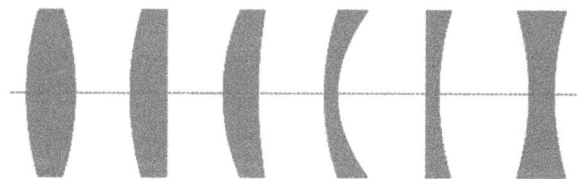

Figure 20.2 There are six different types of lenses: (left to right) biconvex, plano-convex, positive meniscus, negative meniscus, plano-concave, and biconcave.[3]

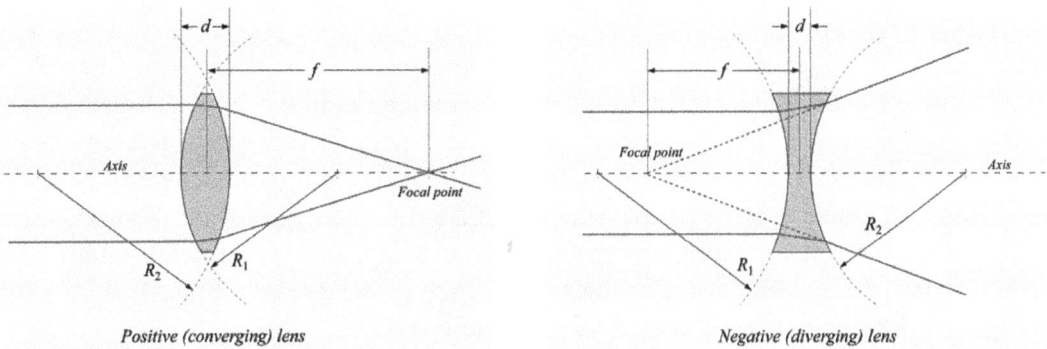

Figure 20.3 A positive (converging) lens (left) and a negative (diverging) lens (right).[4]

acoustic lenses, for example—while the latter spreads light. (Figure 20.3) Lens manufacturers can control the exact amount of power and focal length of a lens by precisely altering the relative curvatures of the two faces.

Light is focused by a positive lens, which means that such a lens magnifies the power of the energy coming through it by taking the light striking over a relatively wide area and redirecting it all into a smaller area—theoretically as small as an infinitesimal point—on the other side of the lens. A lens with a large, blunt focal point only magnifies a little bit, but it magnifies a wider area, while a lens with sharp focal point magnifies more greatly but of a smaller area. (I guess that yin and yang can't help but crop up throughout reality.)

To bring in Tai Chi, finally, this is exactly how fa jing works. In applying fa jing, the Tai Chi Chuanist creates a surge of jing energy, which is essentially a wave of compressed chi supported by correct body alignments and just the right amount of exertion by the sinews and muscles. The wave can be focused either a little and somewhat softly for a non-shocking shove or a lot and sharply for a strike or shocking jolt.

The operation of a negative lens is the yin in action. Or is that reaction? Or non-action? Certainly it's not inaction since something happens. It definitely is the yielding, though, as it takes in, then dissipates, the light, just as the Tai Chi exponent leads an opponent's energy into emptiness either by dissipating the opponent's energy around the sides or by refocusing it somewhere other than the exponent's own center.

Another interesting fact about lenses is that they all have zero thickness. In simplistic and theoretical terms, it's the faces of both sides of the lens—their curvature and relation to one another—that count, not the actual thickness of the lens material. In practice, some lenses have to be thick to accommodate the radical curvatures of the faces, and in such lenses, the faces often have to be shaped in certain ways to account for the thickness of the lens material. But at base, it's just the faces that count. They and their curves are what cause the light to bend from its usually straight line into an alternate straight path, either for focusing or for divergence. In essence, the lens material is just a substrate to hold the faces in place. Lens faces, not their material, are the interface where things happen—where one state transforms into another state—and that interface is infinitely thin even though it does have two sides that are no where parallel.

We tend to think of lenses as clear, curving objects made of glass or plastic. In these objects, the light is bent at the surface of the lens by the difference in refraction between the air and the surface of the material making up the lens, such as glass or plastic. In glass or plastic, this takes place instantly at the curve of the material, but other things or forces can alter the trajectory of incoming light/energy. The aforementioned microwave, electron, and acoustic lenses use different methods to focus the energies they deal with.

One example is the electrostatic lens, which is a device that can focus charged particles, such as electrons. Electron lenses once found use, for example, in the cathode ray tube electron gun that was the principal mechanism in the functioning of old tube TV screens. And most of us probably have heard of gravitational lensing, in which astronomers use the bending of light rays by the powerful magnetic fields around massive stars and galaxies to view magnified images of stars or galaxies that lie great distances beyond.

When you get down to it—and related to Tai Chi in a more direct sense—a rocket motor is really a lens that focuses the tremendous energy of the burning rocket fuel into a relatively narrow but highly intense beam of energy powerful enough to thrust the mass of the spacecraft out of the well of Earth's gravity. The rocket's "focal point" is its ignition point within a constricted space with a narrow outlet. Similar is the way a hose nozzle focuses the energy of a stream of water. Also there are explosive lenses, which are explosive charges shaped to produce a focused blast. Think of a sharply focused expulsion of Peng energy, as in Press. And speaking of blasts, how about those stereo speakers blasting music? Aren't they, in effect, lenses that transform and magnify electrical pulses into conically expanding sound waves?

It's clear that lensing is a basic tool that can be used to act on and manipulate moving energy—be it light, microwaves, burning rocket fuel, water, sound, or a great many other forms of energy. Even chi. In a very real sense, Tai Chi movements operate on physical and energetic levels as lenses that can focus or disperse one's internal energy. At various places along the chi meridians are certain acu-

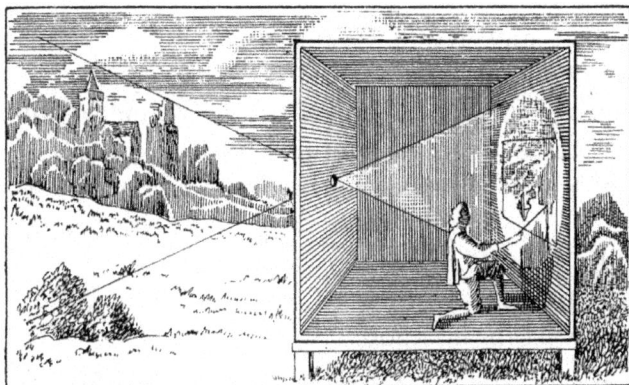

Figure 20.4 Inside a Camera Obscura, an image of the scene on the other side of the wall will be projected through the pin-prick hole onto the wall opposite the hole, but the projection will be upside down and backwards.[5]

puncture points that, because of their locations, can be internally manipulated to restrict or open the flow of chi to create specialized expressions of jing energy.

Three of the more important of these points are the *mingmen* point in the center of the lumbar area which controls the chi flow to the legs through the sacral plexus, the *dazhui* point at the base of the neck which controls the chi flow to the arms through the brachial plexus, and the *daling* point in the inside of the wrist which controls chi flow into the hand and affects the flow in the entire arm. In each case, the power and expression of the chi flow is manipulated to correct effect by how the several acupuncture lenses work together to create various "focal points" and "focal ranges." Both of these are generally articulated by the "terminal" positions of the various Tai Chi postures.

These are examples of chi lensing that take place within the Tai Chi Chuanist's own body, but in practical terms, the entire Tai Chi exponent becomes a lens. He or she accomplishes this by drawing energy—either the exponent's own energy or the opponent's—through the infinitely thin interface between the opponent and the exponent and altering it in ways that aren't always straightforward, dimensionally speaking. Those ways can twist and turn more than one way simultaneously, can expand and contract along curving lines that recoil on themselves, and can use various other deviously sinuous means to subtly defeat an opponent.

The dynamic produced by Tai Chi movements finds a perfect parallel in lenses because a lens doesn't just make things look bigger or smaller; it inverts an image projected through it. (Think: Transforms attack into defeat.) This is what happens inside a Camera Obscura, the earliest practical camera. (Figure 20.4) It consists of a darkened room with a single pin-prick-sized hole in the middle of one wall. Although some historians believe that the Camera Obscura dates back to the Pleistocene, the device first appeared in the historical record in writings of the Chinese sage Mo Tzu dating to about 500 BCE in China.

When you stand inside a Camera Obscura, an image of the scene on the other side of the wall will be projected through the pinprick hole onto the wall opposite the hole, but the projection will be upside down and backwards. Mo Tzu correctly posited that the image is inverted because light travels in straight lines, and his followers developed this into a theory of optics.[1]

Observing illustrations of reality flipped and flopped through a lens, I keep seeing this, in profile, as the infinity twist in the middle of the taijitu. (See "The Infinity Twist," later in this volume.) In other words, because a lens is round, light going through it produces a circular image on a plane parallel to the other side of the lens. But the energy involved—the light itself—is not the flat projection. Instead it fills the space between the lens and the surface with a conical construct of light, of which the flat projection of a Camera Obscura is really just a slice. If the surface on which the image is projected is removed, the conical projection simply travels on infinitely, albeit with steadily diminishing effect with each passing second. At some point, the energy is no longer easily recognizable as a cone, but it is one, nonetheless, just an extremely tenuous one.

Now, let's look at the other side of the lens: the side that is the original reality projected through the lens. Interestingly, because the lens only takes in a circular segment of that reality, the energy of the light involved in the projection also is in a conical shape that is exactly the same size and dimensions as the projection, just in its "normal" orientation instead of inverted. And the reality it expands through also goes on forever.

We can graphically relate this internally energetic double cone shape, with the lens at its pinch point, to the figure-eight at the core of the taijitu. Looking at both figures flat-on, we only have to cap off the ends of the cones with arcs, which far from terminating the energy, simply recycles it back through the resulting infinity symbol. And the parallel continues when one considers that the lens and the central juncture of the taijitu's figure-eight are both interfaces between the yin and the yang—the this and that—where energy going through the focal point turns inside out and backwards.

This idea becomes even more interesting in terms of physical dynamics when one views the linked cones not as a flat figure-eight but as a three-dimensional hour-glass, with each side of the lens projecting the other side equally. In a sense, both cones are sets of reality that are interposed upon each other, though they are flipped and flopped on each side of the lens, creating a dynamic interplay of yin and yang within the double cone shape. Looking at it this way, a lens becomes the neck of an hourglass through which the sands of space-time continuously flow from one state to another and back again. This makes lenses seem like some sort of dimensional leaks that transpose reality into its opposite at an infinitely thin and magical interface. Heck, maybe they are, and we just can't get through.

If all this isn't odd enough, consider the following. Tai Chi Chuanists frequently talk about yin and yang but rarely about the interface between them—between this and that, between order and chaos. After all, true Tai Chi should be able to transform not just the aggression, but the aggressive intent of an opponent, into their opposites. As it is precisely at the lens-like interface between aggression and non-aggression that Tai Chi functions, I thought that it might be edifying as well as educational to observe this interface in action. Could I actually witness "the one" transform into "the other?" Probably not, but you know, I gotta try, I wasn't doing anything else, and there was a magnifying glass right in my desk drawer.

Because of the lens's particular shape, I know that it shows an upright image only when the face of the glass is relatively close to the object that it is magnifying and when my own face also is relatively close to my side of the glass. This brings both the viewed and the viewer within the proper focal range of the lens. But if I hold the magnifier at arm's length and look across the room—or even at relatively close objects—not only are they blurry to one degree or another, they're upside down and backward.

Okay, I expect that, just as I expect proper alignment when I'm using the magnifier within its focal range—close to the object being magnified and close to my face. But we all know that upside-down-and-flopped and right-side-up-and-not-flopped are two diametrically opposed extremes. And both are visible through a glass and theoretically could be viewed sequentially and without interruption. That led me to wonder what I would see if I watched through the magnifier while I gradually changed its distance from both its object of focus and my eyes? Would the actual interface between yin and yang become visible or apparent in some way or other?

At first, I tried that, holding the glass at arm's length while I stared through it at the bulletin board on the wall behind my desk. I could make out a word—properly upright—that was scrawled on a piece of paper tacked there, and I tried to keep the glass trained on the word while I slowly retracted my arm. The scrawled word grew predictably blurry and finally magnified out, so to speak. Only when the glass was very close to my eyes could I again see the bulletin board upright, albeit extremely out of focus. Everything in between the two orientations had been a blur, and I saw—and learned—nothing.

Part of the problem was that I'd changed both the distance between the lens and my eyes and the distance between the lens and the object of observation. That gave me two variables where I required but one. I needed something I could focus on steadily and actually see some sort of image throughout without changing the distance of the magnifier from my eyes. I chose the juncture of the desktop and the strip of bare wall just below the bulletin board. When I held the glass at arm's length, I could see an upside-down image of the juncture, and if I held the glass lower, but still at the same distance, I could see the desktop in its correct, upright position. Somewhere in between was that place where the inverted image changed to the normal image.

I moved the glass slowly down and up many times, each time with the same result: When I lowered the glass, the image of the juncture would move from top to bottom (upside down and backwards), and then, for just the barest of moments, the image would blur out and all visible movement would halt in a sort of haze. Then, as I continued to lower the glass, the image resumed moving as the desktop came into increasing focus, but this time the movement was from bottom to top, or, oriented normally. The interface of yin and yang, chaos and form, upside-down and right-side-up, was in there, but it just couldn't be seen behind the blur of its state of non-formation.

I know that optics experts and so forth will point out that the blurring is because of focal-this and focal-that, and yeah. Okay. But so what? It's also philosophically interesting from other standpoints. I like looking for similarities, parallels, and congruencies, and their opposites, in systems of energetic balance. And I can only say that, with my magnifying glass experiment, I watched as one state of reality devolved into the inchoate haze of non-existence, only to reemerge a moment later as its opposite state of reality. Everything in between remained a mystery.

Something similar to the blurring happens to astronomers who peer into the farthest reaches of the universe. They now have instruments that can observe so far in distance—and therefore, back in time—that they can discern the state of the universe just moments, astronomically speaking, after the Big Bang. The Big Bang is, of course, the lens through which our universe was/is being projected—that pin-prick hole that eventually spread the energy coming through it into a vast area. But even as researchers pierce the veil of time and space more and more deeply in their search for the moment of the Big Bang, all they can see is the increasing haze of radiation that, like a dense fog, eventually hides anything farther and older—and more primordial—from view.

Again, I'd seen nothing, but in this case I did learn something: We probably will never be able to actually witness or discern, either visually or by other means, the interface between the states of yin and yang. Reality is binary, but every thing and every force is a heady mixture of the yin and yang, and any direct view of the division between the two is necessarily obscured in a haze of motion, uncertainty, unformation, and transformation.

Oddly enough, it would seem that when things or forces suddenly transform from one state into the opposite, they, in essence, vanish from reality for a split micro-instant. Reality is, in reality, only energy that is manifesting through motion and binding together, and if the empowering energy ceases to manifest and move, so do its manifestations. When an object moves in one direction and then changes to the other direction, there is a moment of pure equilibrium when the one has not yet changed into the other. A moment in which there is energetic stasis, or non-being. The art of Tai Chi teaches the exponent to avoid this bifurcated state by effectively weaving his or her movement and energy without pause, without loss of momentum or continuity, allowing it to emerge on the other side both coherent and magnified.

For the Tai Chi Chuanist, the art is like a lens. At its best, it can aid in teaching us how to diminish the tensions and magnify the relaxation of our bodies to gain maximum use of them and to both expand and focus our personal energies. In a practical, martial sense, it can teach us how to diminish the power of incoming energy or magnify the effects of seemingly small movements. And because Tai Chi closely adheres to the laws of nature, it also is a lens through which we can view the world and parse the mechanisms and effects of the reality in which we live.

Perhaps that leads to greater power and to a greater understanding of life and the place in which we find ourselves, and maybe it might even be able to shed light on the deeper mysteries of the universe. Those outcomes are for the individual to explore, but in any case, the search sure is interesting.

Pass me that magnifier, will you? It's time to do Tai Chi.

> Where mystery is absent, art is no more than prettiness, or else a mere depiction of an object's gross, tangible quality, whereas, where mystery is sensed, reality is not far off.
>
> —John Blofeld
> *Taoist Mysteries and Magic*

Digging the Vibes

"Good, good, good, good vibrations," sang the Beach Boys back in the day, referring to the good feelings one has in beneficial circumstances. Indeed, the Beat and Hippie cultures of the past century lauded "good vibes" as an excellent condition of life that should be sought and nurtured. And maybe they were on to something. If humans—and indeed, all life-forms—produce a bioelectric field, then such an energy construct must be affected by other such fields and waves of energy, even if the individual is not aware of those effects or is not sensitive enough to perceive them consciously. If so, one would certainly want any impinging energy to be beneficial, not negative.

This brings us to the subject of music and how this art form affects listeners. As with most aspects of reality, music has its own spectrum of listener effect, from the highly intellectual approach of jazz and avant-garde music to the free-form soaring of new age and space music to the beat-heavy impact of pop, rock, and rap. The former group tends to move the mind, the second motivates the spirit, and latter has its greatest effect on the physical level. But in all cases, music is the projection of vibrations toward a listener, and those vibrations necessarily impact not just the eardrums but the body's entire physical construct, including the body's energy field.

Some listeners prefer certain types of music that resonate, perhaps, with their own energetic frequencies, while others explore greater ranges, appreciating the varying effects that different types of music have on them. Most of us probably dislike any music that does not resonate well on any level, and indeed, there are some people who hate music entirely, experiencing it as disturbing noise that grates on their beings.

This idea also begs other questions regarding the impacts that external energy sources have on one's personal energy field. Close to home are the now-ubiquitous and steadily increasing wireless communications we rely on in our daily lives. Although few of these sources are massive, they are pervasive, particularly in urbanized areas. And generated farther from home are gravity waves, postulated by Albert Einstein and now established as fact with the scientific registering of such waves. Gravity has a direct effect on magnetic and electromagnetic fields, so any gravitational wave that passes through Earth's space also will affect all fields on the planet, even our relatively minute human-generated energy envelopes, momentarily distorting them one way or another as the wave passes through.

Because our personal fields are directly tied to our nervous systems and psyches, I'm led to wonder about what effect, if any, that ripples in space-time actually have on whole populations. Surely they would perturb the energy fields of humans on a large scale. I'm sure you've had days where everything goes either right or wrong or you suddenly have unexplained but severe shifts in mood, and when you mention it to others, they respond by saying they've been having an equally good or bad day, too. Are oscillations, whether caused by gravity waves or strong electromagnetic signals, in the general matrix of energy fields that surround us as individuals, our planet, and our solar system somehow responsible for large-scale fluctuations in mood, temperament, excitability, or even sanity, not to mention physiological sensations? In a world gone suddenly crazy in a very short span of time, this is, perhaps, a significant question.

Part V

Toying with Tai Chi

21. Introduction

The movements of Tai Chi Chuan can be difficult to learn, but once you do, they seem perfectly natural as you flow through the form. In fact, being relaxed and natural are the name of the game in Tai Chi, otherwise, playing Tai Chi becomes a chore rather than a relief, and the practice becomes less effective for both health and self-defense. That doesn't mean that Tai Chi should be easy or rote or effortless. It's still work, but work of the sort that elevates rather than crushes. In that respect it has much in common with play. Indeed, practicing Tai Chi often is called "playing Tai Chi."

Children at play instinctively understand that their play is in deadly earnest as long as it remains unattached to outcome. This allows their actions to have meaning without negatively impacting their lives after play. I can be the nasty bad guy in play, but afterwards, I revert to my usual, less bad self. In this essay, though, I'm not going to digress further into play as a topic; instead, in this section, I'm going to look with Tai Chi eyes at some of the objects that children and adults play with and how they illustrate Tai Chi principles.

22. Tops and Gyroscopes

One of the first Tai Chi metaphors I ever heard was a comparison of the Tai Chi Chuanist with a spinning top. There are four basic types of tops: hand-thrown, spindles, device activated, and mechanical. (Figure 22.1) Each type is spun in a different manner, but no matter how a top is fashioned or how it begins spinning, the result is the same: It spins around its axis until friction consumes enough energy for the top to wobble, then fall over.

But while a top is spinning, if an object, say a penny, is tossed at it, the top's spin both diverts and repels the object in the same instant. In part, this occurs because, in the moment that the penny strikes, the spin moves it laterally away from the body of the top, and then that same spin, now lateral for a split instant to the penny's tangent, propels the penny away. But the spin is possible only because the top, when spinning, rotates around an axis. In other words, it embodies Central Equilibrium. Without Central Equilibrium, the energy that can cause spin will only cause uncontrolled tumbling.

Central Equilibrium does not exist in an inert top, even though the object does have one major potential axis and a great, almost infinite, number of other potential axes. It is the rotational movement of the top's mass around one of these axes that generates Central Equilibrium. Central Equilibrium, in other words, does not exist in a body at rest. Without Central Equilibrium, there is no spin, and spin cannot exist without generating a Central Equilibrium.

The idea in Tai Chi is to refine the diameter of Central Equilibrium to an infinitely small axis, around which perfect balance exists. Of course, a Tai Chi Chuanist does not literally spin like a top, but the exponent is trained to rapidly rotate around his or her axis in short to longer arcs, using particular arm and hand movements to engage with, stick to, and control the opponent during the course of the rotation.

Interestingly enough, the stability—call it rootedness—of the top while spinning around its Central Equilibrium also is an equal factor in the top's ability to repel a penny. While a top is spinning, it is impossible to touch its Central Equilibrium because the body of top will repel any touch. Okay, maybe not always, you say. You can toss an anvil on the top and crush it, proving me wrong. But am I wrong? The anvil is massive enough to halt the top's spin in the instant before it crushes the top. So, the spin still has to be halted in order to touch the top's Central Equilibrium, in which case, the Central Equilibrium still is lost and no longer there to be touched.

But I digress, and dropping an anvil onto a top is tantamount to throwing a fully-loaded eighteen-wheeler onto a Tai Chi player. In practical terms, if you nudge a top, your finger will be deflected, and the top might creep backward a bit, but it will remain in a relatively upright orientation. Indeed, you will feel a return pressure if you nudge it. The rootedness of a spinning top might be related to the fact that it is completely single-weighted—its balance is almost absolutely singular. Tai Chi players know that real power is generated from single-weightedness in the body, which allows not only for stability but for full expression of power by combining physical movement with a surge of internal energy, both along a single path.

Gyroscopes take the ideas of Central Equilibrium and single-weightedness a step farther. (Figure 22.2) Once you set a gyroscope

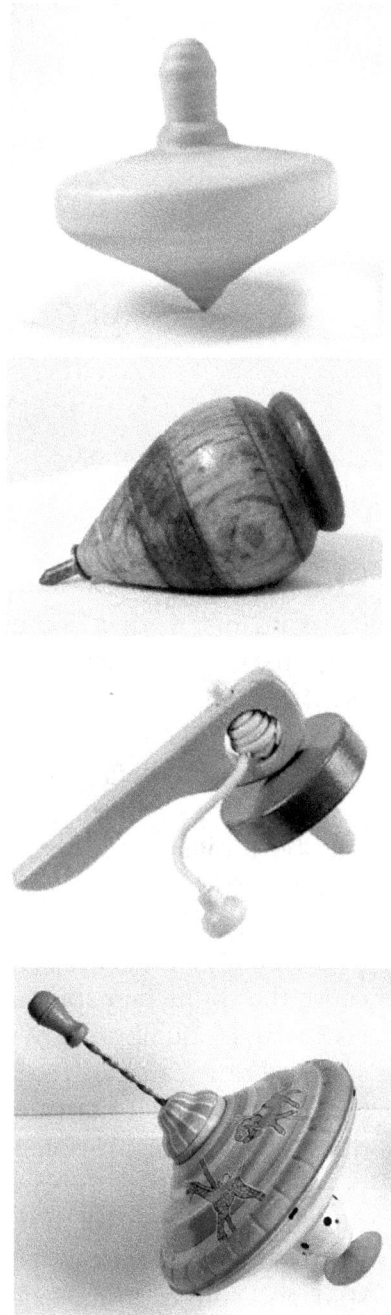

Figure 22.1 Four types of tops, from top to bottom: spindle, hand-thrown, device activated, and mechanical.[1]

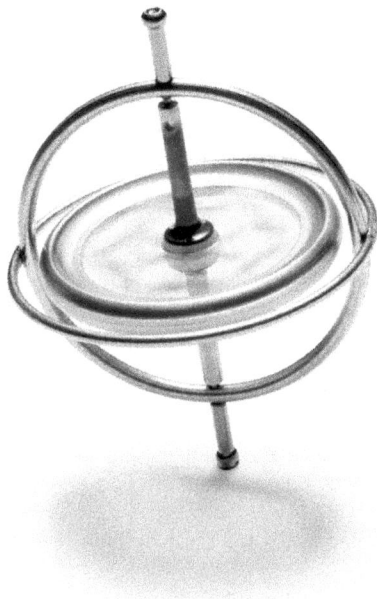

Figure 22.2 A spinning gyroscope exhibits equal weight in all directions lateral to its plane of spin. All the forces are directed into its foot.[3]

spinning, the entire device takes on the quality of a living body that will twist and writhe when you pick it up and handle it. Because of the flywheel-like spin of the rotor, a gyroscope has almost exactly the same weight at every degree of its circumference. And because of this absolute equilibrium throughout the body of the gyroscope—rotor, gimbal, and frame—all the weight of the gyroscope is focused down into its single foot. Remarkably, you can lay a spinning gyroscope almost onto its side, with only its foot touching a pedestal or table edge, and it will seemingly float there, sideways, in apparent contravention of the pull of gravity. Since all the forces of the gyroscope are directed down into the foot, even a canted gyroscope has a Central Equilibrium that roots itself directly to Earth's gravity at the central point of its foot.[2]

In fact, a spinning gyroscope can give a good sense of how rootedness can develop natural resistance—by this I mean internal energy rather than strength—against outside force. Set a gyroscope spinning, place it on its foot, and try giving it a gentle shove from the side with your finger. You'll feel pressure pushing back, even though the gyroscope has neither muscle, motors, nor intent.

The idea of rotation is the keystone of most transcendent symbols: of the mediaeval Rota; of the Wheel of Buddhist transformations; of the zodiacal cycle, of the myth of the Gemini; and of the opus of the alchemists.

—J.E. Cirlot
A Dictionary of Symbols

The Taoists say that if things move in a balance, it is essential that the pivot of this balance should be not a thing but a nothing, which is the transcendent empty of all attributes. Chuang Tzu illustrates this point with his usual humorous profundity:

"The Spirit of the Clouds when passing eastwards through the expanse of Air happened to fall in with the Vital Principle. The latter was slapping his ribs and hopping about; whereupon the Spirit of the Clouds said, 'Who are you, old man, and what are you doing here?'"

"Strolling," replied the Vital Principle, without stopping.

"I want to know something," continued the Spirit of the Clouds.

"Ah!" uttered the Vital Principle, in a tone of disapprobation.

"The relationship of heaven and earth is out of harmony," said the Spirit of the Clouds; "the six influences do not combine and the four seasons are no longer regular. I desire to blend the six influences so as to nourish all living beings. What am I to do?"

"I do not know!"cried the Vital Principle, shaking his head while still slapping his ribs and hopping about. "I do not know."

The six influences mentioned here are the Yin and the Yang, the wind, rain, light, and darkness. The Yang, although invisible, has a positive movement; the Yin is what the Yang moves into, though it has a negative, or seductive, activity of its own. Wind, rain, light, and darkness are phenomena resulting from the complementary movement of the Yin and the Yang. The Vital Principle is not a thing in the usual sense of the word, bur rather that by which we may understand how a process and its products are hopelessly entangled with each other: the All is the One, and its harmony comes by itself.

Chinese philosophy has made great play with the complementary opposites of the Yin and the Yang, taking good care never to give them a status independent of each other. We can see this in the diagram known as the T'ai Chi, a circle formed of two interlocked tadpole shapes of black and white, in which the white tadpole has an eye of black, and the black an eye of white—a figure that says plainly that the positive energy of the Yang still contains something irretrievably negative, and then in the end everything consists of a movement that turns into its opposite.

The T'ai Chi also evades the question of which comes first, the Yin or the Yang, in a way that reminds one of the curious entry at the very beginning of the library catalog in the British Museum: "A. See B. A correspondence between two clergymen on Regeneration and Baptism. (The letters are signed alternately: B., and A.) 1867." For Yang, see Yin: there is no better way of dealing with such opposites than by making them play pingpong with each other, the point being less to win a game than to keep it going for as long as possible.

—Francis Huxley
The Way of the Sacred

23. Drum Monkey

Another amusing toy that is similar in its reliance on Central Equilibrium is what I used to call a twizzle drum until I learned the term "drum monkey," which is much more colorful. (Figure 23.1) It's also more commonly called a hand drum, though lots of small drums that are struck with the hands, such as bongos and tambourines, also are called hand drums.

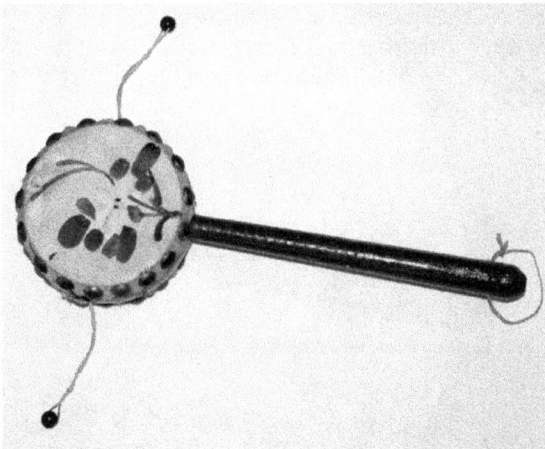

Apparently the drum monkey has no specific origin since it can be found in Asian, African, and Native American cultures. The real use of drum monkeys is ceremonial, though most people think of them as novelty toys. But their import for Tai Chi can be seen during the climactic fight in *Karate Kid II* when the villagers twizzle drum monkeys to encourage Ralph Macchio's character to go with the flow so he can defeat his opponent.

When you look at the action of a drum monkey, it's easy to see the message Macchio's cheerleaders were sending: Loosen and relax your shoulders, and let the

Figure 23.1 Twizzling the handle of a drum monkey will cause the beads on the ends of the strings to slap against the drum heads even though the strings are completely without energy of their own.

twisting of the body around Central Equilibrium (the handle) naturally rotate the drum (the torso), powering the arms and fists (the strings with the beads attached to their ends) in the appropriate directions. After all, a drum monkey has absolutely no strength in its arms, yet the rotation of its body around Central Equilibrium causes the strings and terminal beads to whip quite furiously back and forth against the drum heads. In Tai Chi, one simply uses the legs to powerfully twist the waist, whipping the upper body, which is controlled through refinements of the arm and hand movements to produce desired martial effects.

The interaction implicit in dualism is represented by the famous symbol of the Yang–Yin, a circle divided into two equal sections by a sigmoid line across the diameter, the white section (Yang) having a black spot within it, and the black (Yin) a white spot. These two spots signify that there is always something of the feminine in the masculine and something of the masculine in the feminine. The sigmoid line is a symbol for the movement of communication and serves the purpose of implying the idea of rotation, so imparting a dynamic and complementary character to this bipartite symbol. The law of polarity has been the subject of much thought among Chinese philosophers, who have deduced from this bipolar symbol a series of principles of unquestionable value, which we here transcribe: (a) the quantity of energy distributed throughout the universe is invariable; (b) it consists of the sum of two equal amounts of energy, one positive and active in kind and the other negative and passive; (c) the nature of cosmic phenomena is characterized by the varying proportions of the two modes of energy involved in their creation.

—J.E. Cirlot
A Dictionary of Symbols

24. Rubber Bands

Rubber bands might be the only "toy" that can be found in every office. You can stretch them, shoot them, cat's-cradle them, and twist them. Not only are they fun, they are instructive for Tai Chi.

The way that a twisted rubber band can store energy then release it is amply demonstrated by rubber-band airplanes: those balsa wood toy fliers with red plastic propellers and tiny wheels mounted on springy wires. (Figure 24.1) Twist the propeller for a large number of turns, then let the plane go, and the uncoiling energy of the rubber band spins the prop, which pulls the plane through the air.

Tai Chi, too, relies on twisting movements to coil energy that then uncoils into, against, or away from an opponent. The main difference is that the rubber band in the airplane is twisted for a large number of turns, while the Tai Chi Chuanist only twists part way around. But the elastic bands of the human body—known as ligaments, tendons and fascia—are considerably more powerful than the rubber band in a toy airplane, and the latter two are connected to major muscles and muscle groups. Even a partial twist and recoil of the body, appropriately applied and augmented by proper muscular action, is powerful enough to send the opponent flying. Interestingly, the uncoiling often is accompanied by a corkscrewing movement

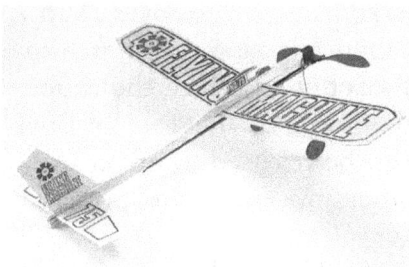

Figure 24.1 Rubber-band balsa airplanes are powered by the twisting of an elastic band that then releases its energy in a coiling movement, driving the plane through the air.[1]

of a limb—usually an arm—that aids in expressing the power of the uncoiling, just as the uncoiling of the rubber band in the airplane activates the corkscrew of the propeller, which is what actually manifests the energy from the coiled rubber band. (See "Natural Patterns" for a discussion of spirals and corkscrewing action.)

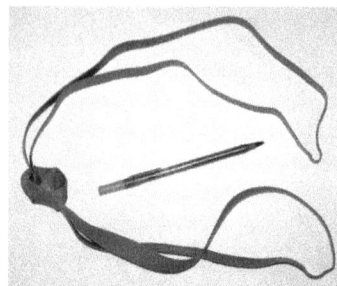

Figure 24.2 My large rubber band. The knot in the middle is to shorten the total length of the band. You could use a bungee cord with its ends hooked and taped together.

Rubber bands can be stretched and released as well as twisted. Who among us hasn't shot a rubber band across the room—probably at somebody? In a very similar way, the Tai Chi player can stretch or compress tendons and fascia, loading them with elastic energy that can be suddenly released against or away from an opponent. Often the energy that is loaded comes from the opponent's own force, which then, in that mysterious interface that exists between yin and yang, is transformed into the exponent's power. Depending on the method of release, the resulting surge of energy can be controlled as a dull wave front that can surgingly expel an opponent, or as a sharp jolt that will penetrate his body.

I have employed a large rubber band in my classes as a teaching tool. It's a big one that I found at an office supply store, and the darn thing cost about $7! (Figure 24.2) You also could also use a bungee cord whose ends have been hooked and duct-taped together. I have the student loop the band around both wrists, for example, and do split movements such as Slant Flying or Single Whip, telling them to feel the growing tension and to control it not through the band but through their shoulders and back. In essence, the rubber band amplifies the elastic stretch and release of the tendons and fascia and gives even a novice a tangible sensation of stretching out and then releasing the stretch instead of simply moving the limbs without internal energy. In effect, the rubber band gives a dynamic sensation of using the elastic power of the Tai Chi Bow. (See later.) In some split movements, the stretch can be released to effect from either end (Slant Flying, for example), while in others, the release is primarily unidirectional (Single Whip, for example).

I've also seen one prominent Tai Chi teacher employ a rubber band as a teaching device. He has his students string the band around their legs at knee height. The band is of a size that it will tighten as the student stretches into Bow Stance. This would give the novice student the tangible sensation of having to press the knees slightly outward to increase stability and rooting.

25. Magnets

Magnets are everywhere, from toy horseshoe magnets to the sun and other celestial bodies. They're found in motors, generators, loudspeakers, electric guitar pickups, computer drives, compasses, and the rubber seal around your refrigerator door—and in the kitschy kitchen magnets you've stuck on the outside of that door. Every electrical wire and device is surrounded by an electromagnetic field, we live totally immersed in the magnetic field generated by Earth, and each of us generates our own magnetic field, albeit a weak one. Magnets are ubiquitous, and they are quite useful as well as being quite natural. Even alone, they make interesting toys as evidenced by the horseshoe magnets you can find in a large number of toy boxes. In fact, electromagnetism is one of the four fundamental forces of nature, along with the strong nuclear force, the weak nuclear force, and gravity. (Many physicists now do not consider gravity to be a fundamental force, but simply the effect of mass warping space-time. Okay. But if I stumble, gravity, whatever it is, will instantly take over and whop me with that mass.)

Most of us know that a magnet generates a field of force called a magnetic field around itself and that it has two poles: positive and negative. (Figure 25.2) There, in a nutshell, is the yin and yang of it. The force of the magnetic field emerges from the positive pole, cycles through the space around the magnet in a toroidal pattern, and reenters the magnet at the negative pole. Magnetic fields do not have boundaries and theoretically extend infinitely outward, though in practical terms, the effects diminish greatly with distance. Also, magnetic fields will pass unimpeded or with only minor diminishment through many—but not all—forms of matter, so they're kind of supernatural in that regard.

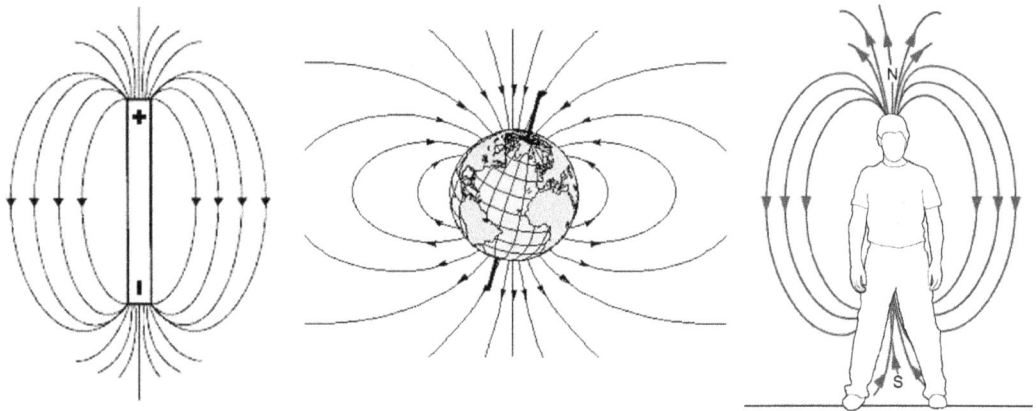

Figure 25.1 Magnetism in a bar magnet (left) is caused by an alignment of the iron atoms in a common direction. Magnetism in Earth (center) is produced by geodynamic processes. The electromagnetic chi field (right) is generated by bioelectric energy flowing along the nerves. The fields of all three objects exhibit polarity and theoretically extend infinitely in all directions but are most powerful in close proximity to the magnetized object.

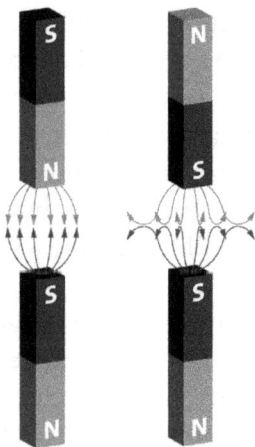

Figure 25.2 Magnets exhibit polarity. Positive and negative are attractive to one another, while positive and positive or negative and negative are mutually repelling.[1]

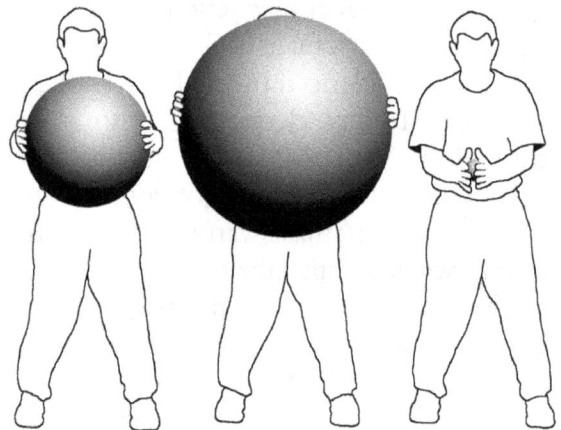

Figure 25.3 The Tai Chi sphere can be played at various diameters. The larger the sphere, the more diffuse the sensation between the hands, while smaller manipulations create a greater sensation of heat and density.

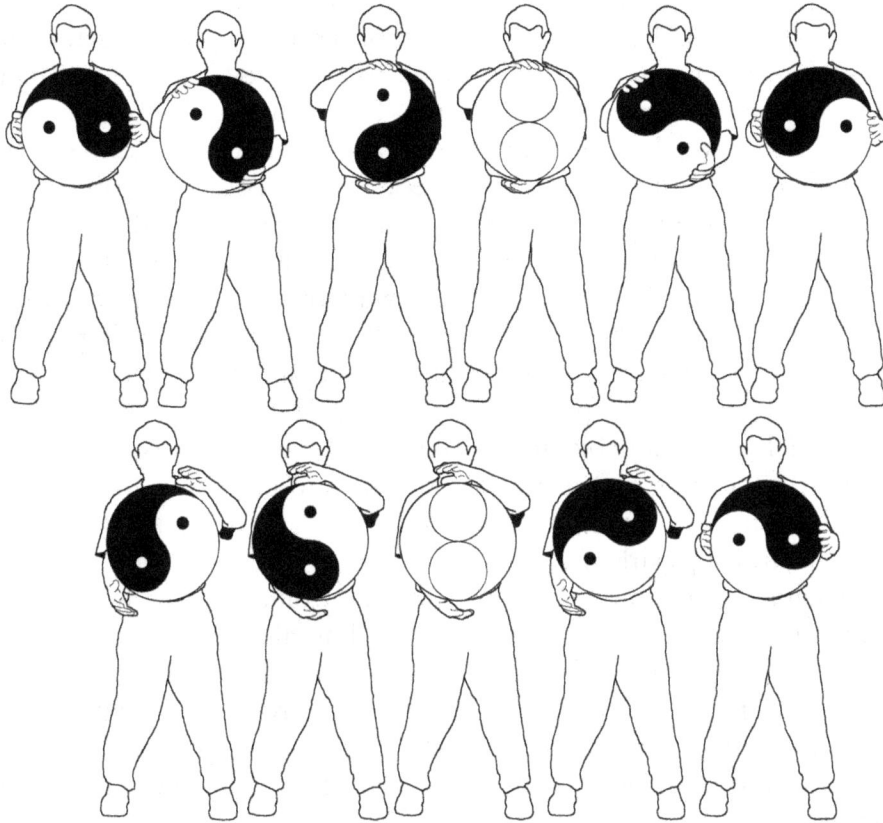

Figure 25.4 The basic Tai Chi manipulation is to roll the Tai Chi sphere from side to side. The spheres with the blank double fish indicate the moment when the energy switches polarity and the ball starts rolling in the opposite direction.

The Eurocentric view of Earth orients the negative pole of planet Earth at the top and the positive pole at the bottom. This is undoubtedly an artifact of the age of European exploration, when the compass was the mariner's major guiding tool. The magnetized needle of a compass points north because the positively charged end of the needle is attracted to the Earth's negative pole, and the Earth's magnetic polarity was not understood at the time. Had it been, we might be adhering to the ancient Chinese view, which was just the opposite and orients the globe with the South Pole at the top. It is probably a more accurate view if we consider the fountaining of energy to go upward and the reabsorption of it to come in from the bottom, as occurs with any magnet, including the human body.

However you look at it, the polarity of magnets demonstrates the yin and yang of things through magnetic attraction and repulsion. If you bring two magnets together at the opposite poles—negative meeting positive—there will be a mutual attraction. (Figure 5.2) But if you bring the magnets together at similar poles—negative to negative or positive to positive—the two magnets will push against each other with invisible force. The former could be considered an example of single-weightedness and cooperation, while the last two might be examples of double-weightedness and the attendant confrontation of energies that results. If you cooperate and blend your energies, you and your opponent become one, but if you meet force with force, only struggle results.

Many Tai Chi folks know how to play with this repelling force when they roll a ball of chi between their hands. (Figure 25.3) What is happening here is that positive chi energy—which is, at its base, electromagnetic in nature—is emerging from both palms. When positive meets positive, the result is repulsion, and this can be felt as a tangible force between the two palms. Using rotating movements of the hips and waist to motivate the arms and hands gives this force the character of a ball, and this ball can be "rolled" in front of the body, creating a controlled swirl in the individual's chi/electromagnetic field. (Figure 25.4) The rotating of the hips not only causes the rolling action, but it also helps power the energy that creates the ball by sending alternating pulses of chi up the legs as you rotate back and forth, amplifying the chi running down the arms and emerging from the palms. The closer the hands roll and the smaller the ball, the greater the pressure between the palms, and the father apart the hands are and the larger the ball, the less the pressure. Again, the power of a magnetic field diminishes over distance.

Cycling

Learning to do Tai Chi is a little like learning to ride a bicycle. In the beginning, you are unstable, you wobble back and forth, and your control is erratic. You make turns by using your arms to twist the handlebars. Your legs, which alternately pump with the ultimate single-weightedness, easily grow tired. And you have to learn to assume a sitting posture that allows your legs to perform the functions of continuous and alternate pushing (rotating yin and yang) while your upper body performs very different, and mostly lateral, functions.

Over time, though, your legs strengthen, and control over your balance improves. Eventually, you no longer use the handlebars to steer around corners, instead using the waist and torso to lean into and out of curves. Of course, Tai Chi discourages leaning, but the similarity here is that both Tai Chi and cycling rely on the waist to command the movement, and even in cycling, the leaning is from the base of the torso rather than being a floppiness at the waist.

And in the end, both activities become so thoroughly ingrained in your movement patterns that you don't have to pay attention to the activity but can simply enjoy the ride—and maybe even learn to perform a few fancy maneuvers.

26. Newton's Cradle

Next, we'll look at Newton's Cradle, also called Collision Balls and Executive Desk Balls. (Figure 26.1) The former name comes from it's creator, Isaac Newton, the middle name is obvious, and the last one comes, presumably, because 1) only executives can afford to waste money on frivolous items that occupy valuable desk space that they're not using because executives do so little real work; 2) executives have so little to do that they have time to play with such frivolities; 3) executives have so little real creativity that they can easily become mesmerized by a simple mechanical device; 4) executives like to give housekeeping staff difficult objects to dust; or 5) executives perpetually study the middle ball which remains static when two end balls are set in motion, demonstrating the chief tactic of the middleman: Do absolutely nothing but transfer something one way or another and reap profits off the efforts and energy of others.

Okay, I'll stop, though it's easy to be cynical these days. Back to Newton's Cradle. This from *Wikipedia*:

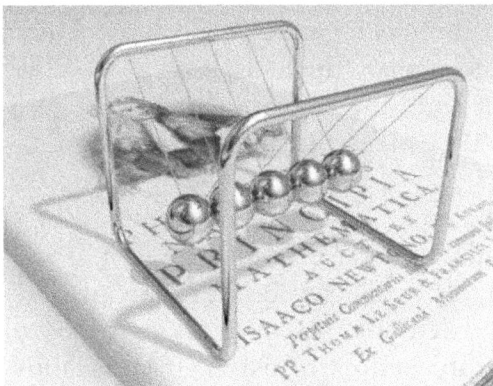

Figure 26.1 Newton's Cradle. If you lift and drop one of the end balls, when it falls and strikes the line of balls, the ball on the opposite end will jump outward. If two balls are lifted and fall, the two opposite balls will jump, leaving the center ball static.[1]

Newton's cradle...is a device that demonstrates conservation of momentum and energy using a series of swinging spheres. When one on the end is lifted and released, it strikes the stationary spheres; a force is transmitted through the stationary spheres and pushes the last one upward.... A typical Newton's cradle consists of a series of identically sized metal balls suspended in a metal frame so that they are just touching each other at rest. Each ball is attached to the frame by two wires of equal length angled away from each other. This restricts the pendulums' movements to the same plane.

If one ball is pulled away and is let to fall, it strikes the first ball in the series and comes to a nearly dead stop. The ball on the opposite side acquires most of the velocity and almost instantly swings in an arc almost as high as the release height of the first ball. [In the absence of friction or other external forces besides gravity, the opposite ball would swing exactly the same height.] This shows that the final ball receives most of the energy and momentum that was in the first ball. The impact produces a compression wave that propagates through the intermediate balls. Any efficiently elastic material such as steel will do this as long as the kinetic energy is temporarily stored as potential energy in the compression of the material rather than being lost as heat.

With two balls dropped, exactly two balls on the opposite side swing out and back. With three balls dropped, three balls will swing back and forth, with the central ball appearing to swing without interruption.[1]

I've quoted the *Wikipedia* entry at length since the presentation was pretty succinct and I'd waste time and clarity paraphrasing it. There's some fancy mathematics involved in the details of the motions of the balls, such as whether or not the balls at rest actually touch or not and other factors that I don't dare attempt to go into. But I think at least one Tai Chi lesson is clear from the motion of Newton's Cradle.

Most of us Tai Chi folks have seen, have demonstrated, or been pushed by a trick Tai Chi application. This is when the demonstrator holds a Press posture and has one person push against his raised arm while several other people line up behind, all pushing, too. As they push, the demonstrator gives a pop of Peng energy from his Press posture, and all the people who are pushing move slightly backward except for the last person in line, who is jolted back farther, often several feet. Clearly this is the same conservation of momentum and energy shown by Newton's Cradle.

In this demonstration, Peng energy can easily be seen propagating through the line of people and finally manifesting in the last person in line. But the more important propagation is less visible because it happens inside the Tai Chi Chuanist's body. We often think of bouncing our energy down into our feet then back up through the legs and torso, into the arms and hands. This movement of internal energy, combined with physical compression and release, acts very similarly to the energy system demonstrated by Newton's Cradle.

At its base, this demonstration recalls the idea from the Tai Chi Classics that one should learn to "pass a thread through the nine-channel pearl." Apparently, the nine-channel pearl was a game in which Chinese girls attempted to push a thread through a ball with nine caddywampus holes drilled in it. In Tai Chi, the nine-channel pearl is the human body, the channels are the major joints that must be aligned correctly to give the exponent's uncoiling force and energy a proper path to follow. The idea is that the Tai Chi Chuanist must learn to push from a single foot and consciously direct the energy sequentially through every joint—ankle, knee, hip, shoulder, elbow, wrist, and the three joints of the phalanges—all the way to the fingertips. When considered like this, Cheng Man-ching advocating the use of Ladylike Wrist during form practice makes perfect sense because that hand form allows the chi to flow unimpeded to the fingertips.

Threading the nine-channel pearl can be thought of as an unfolding process or even a pneumatic process in which the body sort of inflates in a wave that progresses from foot to hand, but in a sense, the dynamics also are similar to those of Newton's Cradle. The joints are like the places where the balls of Newton's Cradle touch, and the body parts are like the balls themselves. Chi in the foot bounces through the ankle joint to the tibia. Then it bounces through the knee joint to the femur, through the hip joint into the pelvis/torso, through the shoulder joint into the humerus, and so forth down the arm and through the last joints of the fingers.

But there is an important difference. In an idealized Newton's Cradle (without friction), the energy propagates through the several balls then knocks the final ball into the air. This ball then falls back with equal velocity, strikes the first of the lined-up balls, and transmits its energy through the line to the ball on the other end. This one reacts by bouncing into the air exactly as high as its initial fall, and so on, each strike imparting only the energy with which it was endowed. The Tai Chi exponent is not so mechanized. The initial impetus of the energy surge, coming either from the opponent or the exponent himself and going down the leg, terminates at the sole of the foot. Because the surface on which the foot rests is solid, the foot, unlike the end ball, has no space into which it can move.

In a way, Earth itself has become the final ball, and clearly Earth is too heavy to move much by pushing your foot down on it. So, instead of swinging out then falling back to retransmit itself back along the path from which it came, the energy instantly rebounds back into the foot. It's as if the energy takes an instantaneous 180° turn inside the Earth, making the foot not just the ball that acts against the ball of the Earth, but also the next ball in line as the energy reemerges into the foot. And because the human body is flexible and mind-directed, the rebounding energy can be tremendously augmented by the strength of the uncoiling leg muscles, tendons, and fascia as it surges up the leg, through the hips and waist, and into the torso.

This augmented energy propagates through the intervening body segments (the balls) and arrives at its terminus (hand, say, but it could be an elbow, shoulder, etc.) in a very powerful state because it has built up momentum and power over a distance of about ten feet—through the body, into the ground, then back up through the body—in a very rapid fashion. So, unlike the end balls in Newton's Cradle, which each receive and transmit exactly the same amount of energy, the end ball in the Tai Chi Chuanist's train of balls—often the hand—receives a seriously amplified pulse of energy that then acts upon the opponent.

In the case of the Tai Chi Peng demonstration describe above, the energy doesn't go all the way through the arm to the fingertips. Instead, it goes only as far as the demonstrator's jolting palm, then through the join between the palm and the inside of the demonstrator's forearm, then through the join between the outside of the demonstrator's forearm and the palms of the first person in the pushing line. Thereafter, each person in line is like a ball that is subsequently jolted through the places where they touch until the jolt terminates, with full force, at the final person in line, who then bounces away.

Maybe we should dub the Peng demonstration outlined above Chang's Cradle, after Chang San-feng.

27. Crack the Whip

Okay, you don't need a toy to play Crack the Whip. But it is play, and this particular game amply demonstrates Tai Chi's whipping power. (Figure 27.1) It's also kind of the yin to the yang of Newton's Cradle: a stretching, flexible, pulling energy rather than a compressive and concussive energy.

For those of you out there who don't know what Crack the Whip is all about, it's when a bunch of kids stand in a line in a big field, sequentially holding hands. Then the person at the head of the line begins hauling backwards, dragging the next person along, who drags the next person, and so forth down the line. Pretty soon, the whole train of kids is snaking around across the surface of the field as the head person turns this way and that, sinuously weaving his followers along behind him.

The pace and turning of the head might appear leisurely and gradual, but as the snaking effect works its way down the line and becomes more sinuous, the people toward the tail end of the line find themselves whipped back and forth as they run along, dragged by the person in front of them. The last person in the line receives the most violent snaking effect and eventually is "cracked" off the end of the line at the apex of a whipping turn and sent rolling and tumbling across the grass. But even as the last person is cracked off and tumbles, the person at the head of the line—the handle of the whip—continues to maintain a leisurely pace. You can see the same sort of effect in bullwhip, of course, but it's also present in other scenarios, such as a roller coaster. The people in the front car experience the most stable ride, while the people in the tail car are more violently whipped and thrown around in their seats

Well, I guess it's time to stop toying around with these ideas and go play Tai Chi. While I might be tempted to think back to my childhood toy box and the Tai Chi toys it held. Instead, I'll try to concentrate on my Tai Chi form, which has become the biggest and best toy box I could imagine. It might be finite in external size—bigger than a breadbox and smaller than a room—but the whole of reality seems to be in there. It's like Felix the Cat's magic bag of tricks or an infinite store where playthings, tools, and insights line the shelves of secrets I didn't even know existed. To discover those secrets, all I have to do is start playing.

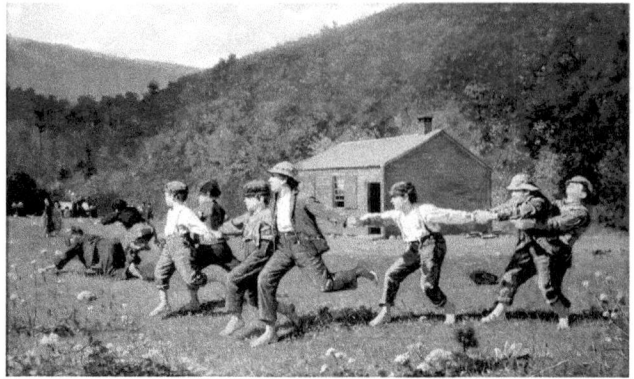

Figure 11 *Snap the Whip,* by Winslow Homer (1872)[1]

I have heard it said that when the level of your personal chi falls below a certain threshold, you expire. This would seem to jibe with the idea that personal chi is a bioelectromagnetic field that, during life, has a higher energetic density that is dissipated at death by entropy.

But a personal field might do more than envelop us with life. In a sense, the personal field might also do something similar to Earth's magnetic field, which protects the surface of the planet from being bombarded with dangerous levels of cosmic radiation. Similarly, the personal field might protect the individual from the constant and pervasive force of the combined fields of the universe—including those of the myriad people around us daily— which, at full force, might overwhelmingly disturb one's energetic being, much like static can drown out a broadcast.

Another interesting offshoot of this is jet lag. Travel lag of any sort might be caused by continuous, prolonged, high-speed movement of a personal field through the universal field, causing a drag, or sort of friction, against one's field, eroding and attenuating it. After all, if it is possible to affect one's personal field with specific exercises and gravity, then other energetic external influences also ought to have an effect on one's field—and sense of well-being—for either the positive or negative. Regarding travel lag, after a short recuperation, the field is regenerated to its former level of strength and one returns to a feeling of normalcy.

Part VI

Principles and Operations

28. Sit Down!

The Tai Chi Classics contain a number of basic rules for Tai Chi, one of the most important of which is to *sung* (song) or to be sung. Sung is a simple word that contains a great deal of import. Most basically, it means to relax the upper body, to sink the sensation of body weight into the lower abdomen and legs, and to coalesce the sensation of the body's internal energy within the lower abdomen. Associated concepts are opening the joints, relaxing the musculature, hollowing the chest, and allowing the arms to droop without being limp. All of these lead one to be able to "settle," which is one of the keys to Tai Chi's martial power. As a concept, sung is easy to understand; however, as a practice, it is very difficult to achieve.

To be able to be sung, one must have proper bodily alignments, otherwise muscles and joints that should be able to relax are busy doing inappropriate work that inhibits the ability to be sung and to circulate internal energy effectively. Improper joint alignment and inappropriate muscular action are defects, and the Tai Chi Classics also encourage us to seek the cause of defects first in the feet and legs—the body's foundation, its stance.

The Tai Chi stance is like sitting on a three-legged stool, although only two of the legs are actual physical legs. The third is Central Equilibrium, which is an axis of the body running from the crown of the head (the *baihui* acupuncture point), through the centers of the tantien and the perineum (the *huiyin* acupuncture point), to the ground. Or, the third leg can be considered an extension of the spine that intersects the ground. Central Equilibrium is the principal stance among Tai Chi's five stances. Or, the third leg can be considered an extension of the spine that intersects the ground. This sensation of possessing a third leg and sitting is present whether one is in horse stance, bow stance, or sitting stance. In all cases, the knees are flexed or bent to some degree.

The deeper the stance, the more of a workout the legs get. However, the depth or height of the stance isn't as much of an issue as are the correct alignments of the body that allow the sensation of sitting to occur. Younger people, as a general rule, have an easier time performing lower stances, and the stances of many Tai Chi practitioners tends to rise with age. But higher stances, aligned correctly, can generate just as much power as lower stances, and often much more rapidly.

> Sung is considered a vital factor in the practice of Tai Chi in that mastery of all the other qualities I have mentioned before depends upon it. Sung can be thought of as the common ingredient among all of those elements. However, to be Sung does not mean that you automatically know how to accomplish these skills. Each task needs its own individual attention for study and practice to acquire, while Sung enhances their development.
>
> —William Ting
> *Essential Concepts of Tai Chi*

The top of the three-legged stool is the pelvic girdle, which is, in essence, a bowl into which the upper body sits. Or should, for sadly that is not always the case regarding human posture. Too often people slump, bend forward at the waist, slouch sideways, or commit other postural errors, all of which cause the muscles of the back and shoulders to perform duties they are not well suited for. This causes undue muscle and joint strain and tension, both of which inhibit chi flow, not to mention making it more difficult to move through one's daily life.

The legs of this three-legged stool can flex and take weight—even the invisible third leg—thanks to proper balance of the upper body on the two tangible legs, which are strengthened in the process. This balance is effected by employing as its base the solidity of the three-faced pyramidal foundation created by the legs of the stool. The stability of this foundation causes the bowl of the pelvic girdle to remain stable, which in turn allows the spine to hold the trunk directly over the pelvic girdle so that the trunk can sit straight down into the pelvis. When the trunk sits into the pelvic girdle, muscles in the back and shoulders that were formerly misused to retain balance can now be freed to effect flexible and loose movement of the trunk.

The sensation of sitting is a prerequisite to the action of sinking or settling flexibly on your legs, which enables you to, in effect, fall down into your stance then surge out of it with a correctly timed push from one leg or the other. This surging rebound is one of the main elements of Tai Chi's martial power. It allows the leg push to accelerate the already existing rebound effect from the settling action, and this, in turn, is given a final impetus by the purely physical unfolding action of the relaxed body. The unfolding produces a whipping action whose snap is a final and appropriate tensing of the whipping body part.

Because the whipping body part is almost completely relaxed until the very brief but very thorough tensing and subsequent instant of impact, and the physical action is one of unfolding, the nerve impulses and accompanying chi fields also whip down the arm in conjunction, only to be halted and accumulated at the appropriate places by the tensing of the body part. From there, the accumulation can be transferred into the body and chi field of the opponent in the same instant that the body part has its direct physical effect. The sharper the physical action, the sharper the chi manifestation. This doesn't mean "greater." A blow bearing a less-powerful emanation of chi will do less damage than a blow of equal physical impact but bearing a heavier emanation.

Relaxation and correct body alignments are absolutely critical in properly effecting movements that work on both the physical and energetic levels. And the basis of those depend completely on the solidity and stability of the body's foundation: the three-legged stool.

And there are other reasons to learn to sit into your pelvic girdle. Tai Chi often is touted as an excellent exercise for aging people. One reason is that Tai Chi's slow movements combined with correct bodily alignments work with but do not stress the weaker muscles and joints in older people. Also, being sunken into your lower body makes you more grounded, so you will fall less, and when you do fall, you will tend to collapse downward instead of toppling and crashing down, resulting in less injury to yourself.

Yet another important aspect concerns the fact that people, as they age, shrink downward from the perpetual force of gravity and bone density loss. Continually positioning your trunk over your pelvic girdle will allow your trunk to settle more naturally and without kinks as you age. This will help prevent stress to the muscles in the back—particularly the lower back—and mitigate pain experienced there.

Any good and valid human practice is built on a good foundation, and Tai Chi is no different. The beauty of Tai Chi is that you can use it to ensure that your own personal foundation is as solid and stable as it can be. Tai Chi's value as a healthful exercise and its martial power are both rooted in a proper stance, so, the next time you stand up to do the form, remember: Sit down!

Following Jing

Tai Chi practitioners recognize that the martial aspect of Tai Chi manifests as jing, or the composite energy that can be produced by the various aspects of chi, sinews, muscles, balance, and other factors all combining in unitary and focused bodily movement. Jing can move relentlessly forward, be released explosively, or be retracted with equally diverse force. There are many types of jing, but one of the most difficult to learn properly is "following jing," or the ability to adhere to an opponent and follow them no matter which way they move or turn. For a hint at the nature of this ability, let's look at the animal kingdom.

It is well established that a tremendous number of animal species can sense and utilize magnetic and electromagnetic fields. Birds often use their sense of place within Earth's magnetic field to direct their mass migrations over distances of thousands of miles. Bats use the same sense to find their way back to their home roosts. Wasps often are drawn to and congregate in large numbers around antenna arrays and microwave relays atop buildings and tall towers.

One of the most remarkable displays of following can be seen in the movements of large flocks of birds and schools of fish as they follow their leaders in flowing, synchronized movements through their environments. One moves, and all the rest spontaneously and instantaneously follow in a way that makes it seem that there are no individuals, only large, flowing, formless creatures composed of many similar parts. Perhaps this sort of movement is the result of the biofield of each individual in these flocks and schools always seeking to find comfortable, natural alignment with those of their neighbors. The result is that the numerous individual fields find themselves part of a gestalt field to which the individuals subsume their wills, becoming, in essence, mere elements, or cells, within massive and unified but essentially amorphous creatures held together by the commonality and alignments of their fields.

Following jing, then, while undoubtedly having a physical component that effects actual physical movement, also has a more critical underlying component whose nature lies in alignment of the practitioner's personal field with the energetic emanations of the opponent. In essence, the practitioner allows himself to be subsumed to the energetic movements of the opponent while not allowing the opponent's movements to result in a direct impact or breaking away.

29. The Speed You Need

Ask the average person what most characterizes Tai Chi Chuan, and they will undoubtedly say: "Slowness." If you spot someone or a group of people in a park, on the beach, or anywhere else, who are slowly waving their arms in arcane patterns and taking measured, deliberate steps, you can pretty much bet they're doing Tai Chi. (We'll except the tragic and all-too-large population of homeless schizophrenics, who also make arcane gestures in parks and elsewhere, following impulses only they can feel.)

The fact that you move slowly during Tai Chi practice has engendered misconceptions—and jokes made on those misconceptions. Indeed, a lot of people, deceived by the slowness, think of Tai Chi strictly as a meditational exercise form and don't realize that it is a very effective martial art. The main misconception regarding its use as a martial art is highlighted by something told to me by one of my students, Dave Walker. (Student is really a misnomer since now he's at least as good at Tai Chi as I am.)

As a young man many years ago, Dave joined Yang's Shaolin Kung Fu Academy in Houston, which was then probably the single-best kung fu school in the area. This isn't to say that there weren't other excellent and knowledgeable teachers and schools around there, a couple of them of much longer tenure. But Yang's Shaolin Kung Fu Academy's director, Jeff Bolt, was a high-level student of Yang Jwing-ming, who, for those unfamiliar with him, was named by *Inside Kung Fu* magazine as one of the ten most-important kung fu figures of the past century.

Dave came to Jeff's school after a few years of taking Taekwondo and karate, and when he first asked Jeff what style of kung fu he should learn, Jeff told him, "Tai Chi." Dave has a stocky body with a naturally low center of gravity that lends itself perfectly to Tai Chi. But when Dave first saw people practicing the Yang Style form, he couldn't figure out how anyone could fight so slowly and yet prevail. Besides, this was the decade of Bruce Lee and the burgeoning of interest in flashier, more energetic external styles, which appeal to young people who have sufficient flexibility and greater energy to burn. So Dave learned Shaolin Long Fist instead.

Dave quit practicing with Jeff's group after a few years, and he had no more form(al) training until he and I met around 2000. He expressed an interest in learning Tai Chi, having come to realize over the years that, while you practice Tai Chi slowly, you learn to be able to use it at any speed you need. With his martial arts background, he learned the long form readily. And he practices it slowly, though his execution can be blindingly fast.

The jokes based on the misconception about practice speed can be pretty funny. There was the guy who came home late, and when his wife asked where he'd been, he said he'd stopped to watch three guys attempt to mug a Tai Chi expert. "I'd have been later if I'd stayed around for the whole fight, but it was taking too long, so I came on home." And then there are humorous *YouTube* videos showing Tai Chi guys mock fighting—including reactions and appropriately pained facial expressions—in very slow motion.

As Dave learned, there are several good reasons to practice Tai Chi slowly, all interlinked and codependent, yet all independently significant. First we'll look at basic physical issues. Tai chi is physical exercise as much as it is martial technique or an internal energy enhancer, and it produces definite physical effects. Foremost among the more obvious of these, not counting martial ability, is enhanced stability.

Stability has a couple of major components: balance and leg strength. These two go hand-in-hand. Proper balance obviously requires greater leg strength, but the fact that greater leg strength is fostered by proper balance isn't as obvious. Improper balance, which is due to incorrect physical alignments, tends to take some of the pressure of standing off of the legs and put it into the muscles and tendons of the back, abdomen, shoulders, and neck, creating a great deal of unnecessary upper body tension as well as instability. The legs become little more than stiff crutches that prop up a stressed-out torso.

Standing with better body alignments allows all of one's body weight to sink straight down into the legs, hence, there is greater involvement of the leg muscles and, as a result, greater pressure on the soles of the feet. Over time, moving through the form with correct body alignments that reposition the weight of the body directly over and straight down into the pelvis strengthens the legs and feet. As with any leg exercise, this can make your thigh muscles—and the tendons connecting those muscles to your knee—achy, especially in the beginning. I've even heard some people complain that doing Tai Chi or chi kung makes the soles of their feet sore. Perhaps, but the payoff is lessened upper body stress and pain and a more comfortable, stable posture. I've experienced all of these leg and sole pains myself at one time or another, but they tend to diminish or vanish entirely. Tai Chi might look relaxed and easy, but that doesn't mean it never brings discomfort. It is exercise, after all. You just make a peaceful face like it doesn't hurt or otherwise stress you out: "My god, what move comes next? I've forgotten what move comes next!"

Tai Chi imparts both leg strength and balance through its stances and in the way it moves without pause between the postures. Throughout all of these postures and movements, one should retain a sense of sitting flexibly rather than being propped up by two rigidly supporting legs, as just described. In these stances, you flex the knees and lower your sense of weight into the posture, predominantly onto one or the other leg so as not to commit the fault of double-weightedness, always with a sense of sitting. A lowered stance promotes a combined sinking and relaxing sensation—sung—that further increases stability. Stances such as this, supporting correct upper body alignments, put the main work of holding up the body onto the muscles and tendons of the thighs, strengthening them and giving the legs a flexible, springing strength in addition to better balance.

Balance goes along with proper body alignments because balance is a product of proper body alignments. As one learns to correctly position one's upper body over a pelvis supported by a sitting stance itself supported by strong leg muscles, balance naturally accrues. And as greater balance is achieved, turning of the body tends to generate, instead of a feeling of being unbalanced or wobbly, the sensation of Central Equilibrium, which is nothing more than an axis of rotation centered on an infinitely small axis running through the core of your body. The more refined one's center of balance, the tighter the radius of rotation of Central Equilibrium. A tighter radius produces greater, faster, and at the same time, more hidden martial effect.

When you first learn Tai Chi, it is difficult to maintain the correct upper body positioning over the pelvis while sinking the postures into the weighted leg. In the beginning, it can only be accomplished by moving slowly and making adjustments over time to your alignments. For example, one learns of the importance of the correct alignment created by slightly tucking the buttocks inward. This causes the tip of the coccyx (tailbone) to point slightly forward.

There are many reasons to do this, but one of the foremost in relation to stability is that you can uses this pointing action when moving from sitting stance into a bow stance—as you might during Brush Knee Twist Step—to help sink and root yourself, even in the midst of movement. You do this by imaging an elastic band strung between the forward-pointing tip of the coccyx and the back of your forward heel. This elastic band contracts as you move from the sitting stance into the bow stance, tending to make you sink and sit into the forward leg in a very stable way instead of onto it in a manner that will potentially overbalance you over your forward foot. Likewise, in sitting stance, the tailbone points at the heel of the weighted leg like it's elastically pulled toward it.

Related to moving forward and backward from leg to leg are Tai Chi's stepping patterns, which encourage intentional placement of the feet to take advantage of geometrically stable angles and relationships between the feet. Over time, these stepping patterns become internalized and instinctual, and when they are added to increased leg strength and improved alignments and balance, they lead to even greater stability. And again, the results can be achieved, at least in the beginning, only through slow, deliberate practice that allows one to find the optimum placement of the feet and, over time, to ingrain that stepping pattern into one's habitual movements.

One positive effect of possessing greater stability is that if you do fall, you're more likely to collapse rather than crash down. This is a version of Tai Chi's principle of folding and unfolding—mostly folding, in the case of falling—instead of rigidly resisting. An even more important result is that stances that sink produce a sensation of rooting one's energy into the ground, lending even greater stability. For this, don't think of tendrils snaking downward from the soles of your feet like tree roots. Visualize the sphere of your chi field—your biofield—embedding itself in the Earth's magnetic field and extending downward, below the surface of the ground—as it actually does. This will produce a sensation of energy expanding out of your feet and into the ground, but this is because the soles of your feet are the only tangible contact with the surface on which you stand, so you tend to feel the energy below them as conical shafts rather than as segments of a spherical field.

All of these effects are possible only because of slow, deliberate movements that train one's instinctual response in an organized and efficient manner to produce results that, over time, are internalized in one's daily movement patterns. As this happens, the movements can grow increasingly fast when used martially, but even then, because the body has been trained slowly and deliberately, the operational principles remain based on relaxation, not on muscular contraction. Tai Chi exercises the musculature in a very limited sense, predominantly relegating the use of it to the lower body—legs, hips, and waist—leaving the torso, arms, and neck relatively free of overt muscular exertion.

Instead, Tai Chi exercises the combined system of ligaments, tendons, and fascia. Ligaments connect bone to bone, tendons connect muscle to bone, and fascia are long—and sometimes broad—sheaves or sheets of tendon material that connect muscle groups. If you've ever seen Body Worlds, the world-famous traveling exposition of skinned and plasticized bodies, both human and animal, the fascia are those long yellow-white structures that overlay and send runners into the major muscles.

In doing Tai Chi, one attempts to motivate upper body motion through deliberate use of fascia and tendons, adding only enough muscular strength to cap off the movement. Tai Chi often is touted as an elixir of health that imparts longevity. One of the main reasons it seems to do this is that Tai Chi constantly exercises the tendon system, extending, compressing, and twisting the ligaments, tendons, and fascia so that they remain flexible. In most older people, the tendons and fascia have lost their flexibility, causing physical rigidity and lack of mobility. Tai Chi's constant expansion and contraction of the tendons and fascia, on the other hand, imparts practitioners with more youthful movements, even into advancing age. A Tai Chi Chuanist's movements produce the exact opposite of the image of the aged person as stiff and tottering. Tai Chi Chuanists aren't necessarily "younger than their age," they just move that way.

Training one's body to move using the tendons and fascia is impossible to accomplish, at least initially, by practicing with fast movement because fast movement, unless trained correctly, will be exclusively muscular and will not be able to properly engage the fascia. Only slow movement can allow a person to relax the muscles enough to train the fascia and tendons to take over. Gradually, after a period of slow training that thoroughly integrates the entirety of the movement as efficiently as possible, the body learns to use the fascia and tendons instinctively, and at that point, extremely rapid—and precise—movement without muscular tension becomes possible. You can even practice the form at faster speeds without tension and to definite benefit.

Perfecting all the physical aspects of Tai Chi—or attempting to!—requires slowness to allow one to move through the postures with a sensation of sitting, to develop correct alignments, and so forth, but these physical adjustments are not possible without Tai Chi's mental aspects, which also require slowness in training.

The first principal mental aspect is observational awareness. This isn't thinking about what you should be doing during a movement, though that is important, but observing how you are doing it, how it feels inside. In other words, you don't just do the movement, you pay attention to how the movement feels and what it does. You observe your stability and balance and how your stance and alignments affect those. You observe your breathing and how and where you are holding tension. And you observe the running thoughts of your ego mind without latching onto them. Observing in this way allows you to turn attention into intention without the intermediary of secondary purpose (conscious/deliberate thought) and without motivating movement with stress, both of which produce exclusively muscular action. (See the next chapter for more on attention and intention.)

> Moving in slow motion enables you to consciously and deliberately access how your mind, body, and energy work. It gives you the needed time to accurately perceive and comprehend the full ramifications of what you are experiencing as you do the tai chi form.
>
> —Bruce Frantzis
> *The Big Book of Tai Chi*

Instead, you learn to motivate movement with mental impulses based on intention alone. And this brings up the second principal mental aspect. Chi, the Tai Chi Classics proclaim, is motivated by the mind. Indeed, Chi is, I believe, the electromagnetic surges that accompany bioelectrical pulses running along the nerves, and as such, it is under direct and immediate control of the mental processes. Muscular action is, as well, but there is a difference. A pulse of chi, being a force that moves concurrently with a nerve impulse, can have an almost instantaneous effect—even while the nerves are only just firing the signals to the muscles to do their biochemical magic of contracting and stretching. This pulse of chi has a pneumatic feel to it and tends to initiate movement in a loose limb without the need to use much muscle. It's almost as if the limb is instantly inflated like a balloon—or even better, an airbag. By the time you need a little muscle to complete the movement, the nerve impulse has finally activated the muscles involved, bringing them into play.

The idea is that you can think a movement, and it happens, though this thinking is not necessarily a conscious process. A fighter who relies on conscious thought will lose because conscious thought is too slow. Instead, training the body with slow movements builds in an instinctual response that can produce movement that is more accurate as well as far more rapid than thinking can accomplish. At the same time, like conscious thought, it pushes electrical signals back and forth in the body, surging chi with each pulse. It is this chi that you attempt to amplify, not the muscular contractions or expansions of a limb.

It's a no-brainer that moving slowly is physically more difficult than moving fast. For any given movement, slow speeds increase the duration of muscular exertion, particularly on the legs, and the length of time in which one must maintain balance. And you're trying to do all that gracefully while keeping a straight face. But it's very much a brainer that moving slowly also is more difficult on a mental level. It's mentally challenging to move slowly. Your mind always wants you to speed up your movements, but you control that desire enough to maintain a steady pace. In the process, you strengthen your will power and the powers of your observational awareness. During that slow pace, you further control the desire to move fast by working to calm any nervous tension or kinks in your muscles or joints that, uncorrected, would tend to impede the thoroughness of a movement.

And you work to calm your mind. If you take one second to do one movement, and you think ten thoughts in that second, then if you take ten seconds to do the same movement, you'll think a hundred thoughts. As each thought has the potential to snatch your attention away from the form, going slowly makes concentration more difficult since you're having to ignore an exponentially greater number of mental distractions as you walk through the postures. If you allow your mind to latch onto these thoughts, you might end up seeing the whole world flash in front of your eyes!

It is practically impossible to completely shut off one's mental blather, but the idea is that you can choose to not let yourself become attached to the thoughts running through your head. They can become like the background sound of surf to those who live by the sea, always present but rarely noticed. And in the end, the control one gains over the body and mind produce another positive effect: greater emotional control. This is bolstered by the fact that Tai Chi trains one to have some degree of martial capabilities, which tends to empower most people and make them more confident and aware of their surroundings and other people.

Over all, moving slowly lends one greater control over one's body, mind, and emotions, all in conjunction. This is the secret of Tai Chi's superiority as a martial art, not its techniques, many of which are shared by numerous external martial styles. The Tai Chi exponent does not rely on techniques to defeat an opponent, though techniques might be used. Instead, the Tai Chi exponent uses a thorough knowledge of self-control gained through slow practice to develop the ability to control others. It is said that Yang Lu-chan was known as the Invincible Yang because he could not be defeated, yet he never seriously injured an opponent—though often they were definitely trying to injure him. That is a perfect example of the nature of the self-control and potential control over others fostered by Tai Chi's slow and deliberate practice.

And that leads us into situational reasons to perform the Tai Chi set slowly. Most of us have heard Newton's Third Law of Motion which basically states that for every action, there is an equal and opposite reaction. The idea is that the more you push against an object, the more you create a counter-movement—such as you also pushing away from the object or feeling a rebound or recoil of some sort —that is of exactly the same force as your push. This illustrates the yin and yang of movement, but the same idea can be applied to slowness and speed: With time, the slower you go during practice, the faster you can go during usage.

This might seem counter-intuitive. Many hard styles of martial arts believe in always practicing at full speed in order to train what might be called a "speed reflex." If you don't practicing hitting fast and hard, they say, you won't be able to hit fast and hard when you need to. But if you practice fast and hard and have not perfected and internalized the proper and complete flow of the movement, the fast movement might actually have defects and blockages that inhibit it from fully carrying out its task quickly, powerfully, and efficiently. And then these defects and blockages get built into the speed reflex like flaws in an otherwise perfect diamond, making it brittle.

Tai Chi takes another approach by using softness, slowness, and deliberateness during practice to set up the proper body alignments and energy channels that will produce an optimum punch, redirection, or other sort of offensive or defensive move. With those alignments in place, all that is then required is to unfold or fold the physical body appropriately while simultaneously pulsing a wave of chi energy in tandem with the physical movement. Both movement and energy are focused at the instant of effect—impact or pull, say. In the case of impact, while the shock of the physical impact will remain generally localized, the chi wave will continue on to penetrate the area, causing further disruption inside the opponent. In the case of pulling or some other yin usage, the physical pull terminates, but the chi wave continues to move away from the opponent for a short distance, carrying the opponent along with it something like a slipstream or undertow might.

In fact, Tai Chi's slowness also improves the speed of a punch in that not only is the punch itself more rapid, it can be delivered at relatively close range and with a seemingly short wind-up. Instead of using a wind-up that draws back then launches forward, Tai Chi employs a spiraling that can be very tight and fast, bouncing the energy from the waist, into the foot, then back up into the body and through the arm to the fist in an instant. This produces a virtual wind-up of eight or ten feet that can impact at very fast speeds in the space of just a few inches. This action is possible because the Tai Chi exponent has done the movements slowly and carefully, observing balance, alignments, application of force, and all the other elements that go into a martial art and exercise form. Also, the slowness of the movements has helped develop the leg muscles and tendons, imparting a springiness. Even more, the exponent has striven to perfect these elements and integrate them into his or her natural movement patterns, and then, at slow speeds, applied observational awareness over time to further polish them and improve the outcome.

Moving slowly is an extremely effective way to train deep and instinctual muscle memory, but it requires a companion component to truly give Tai Chi its Grand Ultimate effects. That companion component is Tai Chi's other defining characteristic, which is one that most people see but don't really notice beyond being able to say that Tai Chi is graceful. Tai Chi is graceful not so much because it is slow but because it expresses continuity.

At its basic, continuity can be defined as connections between sequential events. In Tai Chi, continuity begins on a small scale with the smoothness of individual movements. The Tai Chi Classics state that one should strive to eliminate "projections" and "hollows" in one's movements. This means, simply, trying to move through the postures and transitions without jerkiness, hesitations, weaknesses, or imbalance. Of course, these will always be there, somewhere in the form, even for great masters. After all, we live in a reality in which absolute perfection is not possible. But striving for perfection is still an admirable goal, and great masters are great masters because they have smoothed their projections and hollows to such an extent that they are invisible to most observers.

Over time, the Tai Chi exponent continually strives to smooth the projections and hollows into a steady, continuous movement expressed in unwavering curvilinear patterns. You just can't achieve this by starting with rapid movement. You have to go slowly and with relaxation because, at fast speeds, you are not able to use observational awareness to see or feel your mistakes, and you'll gloss over the jerkiness or slur your movements or otherwise err. In doing so, your habitual practice, which should strive toward perfection, instead will build the error into your movement patterns.

The next level of continuity is that one should progress through the form at an even pace, each posture moving at a steady speed, without hesitation or break in the flow of energy, into the next. Usually in Tai Chi, this pace is leisurely, though once one understands the movements through slowness, it is useful to sometimes practice the form at faster speeds, or to speed up or slow down, because those reveal information about the movements that might be masked by practicing only at a slow pace. Moving slowly through the postures, connecting one set of smooth movements with the next and so on in a steady progression through the form, also trains the body to shift directions and actions as a functional unit, efficiently and without tension, so that if and when the time comes to use the movements rapidly, the body simply reacts as a unit according to the situation.

Steady pacing also has its mental aspect, for it can be a mental challenge to maintain a steady pace throughout the form. There is that already-mentioned urge to constantly speed up that must be conquered. Patience and perseverance are parts of the mental exercise imparted by Tai Chi.

Just as smoothness helps engender pacing, pacing engenders the larger-scale effect of flow. This flow has various elements, all of which become unified and integrated: the sensation of chi flowing or pulsing through the torso and limbs, the sensation of the flow of one's own larger chi field as felt by the moving limbs, and the sensation of external chi fields as felt by one's own chi field and skin. These external fields can be the overwhelming magnetic field of the Earth, the lesser biofields of other people and animals, and even electromagnetic fields produced by electrical devices, wiring, and machinery. The sad truth for those of us living with modern technology—from wiring to machinery to electronic communication devices and equipment—is that the electromagnetic fields and pulses they produce often can have a tangible and disruptive effect on human biofields.

Many people like to go out to the country to relax and feel refreshed. They comment on how fresh the air is, how quite things are, how relaxing the scenery is, and how dark the nights are without all those electric lights shining all the time. Each of these elements has positive effects, but there is another, more subtle, reason. In an urban environment, biofields—chi fields—are constantly being bombarded and permeated and agitated not just by naturally produced magnetic and electromagnetic fields but by what amounts to millions of human-generated electromagnetic signals at any given moment. Most of those human-generated fields, though, are relatively short-range signals that become imperceptible once farther away, such as at a remote beach or forest or mountaintop. No wonder we feel better in places like those.

Moving slowly gives one the opportunity to relax one's body, and once that's relaxed, to use awareness to observe and sense the circulation of internal energy. This will lead to techniques to augment that energy and impart conscious control over it. And in the doing, one also gains greater awareness of the impact that external energy—positive and negative—has on one's being. Just as awareness of chi flow leads to control of that flow, awareness of the impact of external energy can lead one to be able to deal with it in beneficial ways. For positive energy, this might be learning to absorb it rather than to reject it out of fear or ignorance. For negative energy, it might be learning to shunt it aside or otherwise deal with it without absorbing it or trying to shove back at it—a strategy that often leads to escalation of the negativity.

Regarding negative energy on a purely physical level—as with an attack—this means redirecting incoming negative force instead of being impacted by it. But the same principle works on intellectual and emotional levels, too. The key is to not allow oneself to become involved in or attached to the negativity, but to try to lead it into emptiness where it has nothing upon which to act. One response to a verbal attack is to argue back, but another is to shrug and turn away. For a practical emotional equivalent, try suspending a pillow with one hand and punching it with the other. That's antagonism meeting emptiness.

And finally, make what you will of these tidbits relating to physics:

The faster that something goes, the less it weighs. Therefore, up to a point, the slower something moves, the more it weighs. Think about the differences in weight of a conscious person, who has internal movement even if they are inert, and an unconscious one. We sometimes refer to the increased sensation of weight in the latter as "dead weight." Perhaps something like this contributes to the greater sensation of resistance—physical and mental—one feels when moving slowly.

Then there is the law of physics that states that you cannot simultaneously measure both the mass of a particle and its velocity. This indicates that mass and velocity are two sides of the same yin/yang coin. It also implies that using strength (mass) is a more static and less energetically powerful a strategy than using precisely applied movement (velocity) that carries an energetic charge to defeat an opponent.

And last, consider the time dilation that would be experienced by spacefarers traveling near the speed of light. Time becomes subjective for them, and days or weeks or even more lengths of objective time can pass for every hour they travel. This fact has been used to good effect in some science-fiction, though it is more often ignored or circumvented. But there is a Tai Chi—and life—lesson in it: Rapid movement causes you to miss all the details, and as every sage knows, it's the journey, not the destination, that counts.

> Enlightenment has to be won by great and sustained effort; neither divinities nor safes have the poser to bestow it; attainment or failure rest squarely with each individual.
>
> —John Blofeld
> *Taoism: The Road to Immortality*

Abdominal Breathing

When I was four or five years old, I noticed something about the way I was breathing that was different from the way adults breathed. When I inhaled, my stomach expanded, and it contracted again when I exhaled. But the adults I observed breathed differently, expanding and contracting their chests.

I must be doing it wrong, I reasoned. I deliberately started breathing from my chest and continued to do so as I grew up and grew older. Eventually, the episode faded from my consciousness, to resurface only after I took up Tai Chi at age twenty-nine, when I realized what a mistake I'd made. Infants and young children utilize abdominal breathing, but as individuals age, the action of breathing tends to migrate from the diaphragm to the intercostal muscles of the chest, resulting in breathing isolated from the lower lungs. This causes two major, interlinked difficulties.

One is what is referred to as "floating chi," or chi that remains high in the chest rather than sinking into the tantien. Floating chi indicates a lack of connection between the upper and lower body, which results in uncoordinated movement and isolation of body parts during movement. It also can contribute to excitability, over-stimulated emotions, and other issues related to uncontrolled and ungrounded energy.

The second difficulty is that chest breathing does not produce the kind of mechanical stimulation of the tantien required to generate large flows and pulses of chi. This kind of mechanical stimulation is provided only by abdominal breathing in which the diaphragm rhythmically presses downward on the viscera. (See my book, *The Wellspring: An Inquiry into the Nature of Chi*, for a full explanation.)

It took me a number of years to relax again into abdominal breathing, and as I did, I came to understand how vital this form of breathing is to the generation and mobilization of chi. And it also settles the emotions and spirit. Now I sometimes think that the practice of abdominal breathing should be added to the Pre-K and kindergarten curriculums so that young children do not lose this gift. If everybody had greater control of their breathing—and their minds and emotions—we might have a better world.

30. Attention and Intention in Tai Chi Chuan

When I took up Tai Chi Chuan early in 1980, I was looking for a substantial exercise to supplant the calisthenics and yoga-like exercises I'd been doing for several years. The fact was, though these exercises kept me buff and strong, they'd grown boring. I wanted something with more dimension—something, to quote Donovan, "to please my mind as well as my time." I also was interested in something that would impart some self-defense.

This was during the first burgeoning of the modern martial arts in America. Bruce Lee had electrified the screen, the Kung Fu series put Kwai Chang Caine right into our living rooms, and students were flocking to dojos, kwoons, gyms, and parks to practice some kind of martial art. Tai Chi was a popular choice, in large part because its meditative aspects had been fastened on by the New Age movement. A karateka I knew recommended it when I asked his advice about which martial art to take. "It gets better with age," he told me. I knew I would only get older, so that seemed a reasonable lure, and I began attending classes.

Luckily I did choose Tai Chi instead of some harder martial art, though I have briefly practiced a couple of harder styles. From my observations over the past forty years, too many of the harder styles engage primarily in simple rote muscle memory—exactly the mindset I was trying to get away from. Tai Chi, while it does have that aspect, has exceeded my expectations in being as interesting as it is physically worthwhile. I say, "exceed my expectations," because Tai Chi has delivered answers not only to the questions I had, but to questions I didn't know enough to ask.

So, while I would never say that Tai Chi is the "best" martial art, I've found that it's the best for me. And the reason for that is that Tai Chi possesses multifold mental aspects, only some of which are related to the obvious intellectual aspects of Tai Chi, such as the study of Tai Chi history, philosophy, precepts, methodology, and so forth, or trying to understand the literalness of the form and its movements. More important to the practice of the art are the mental aspects of attention and intention. I didn't know about these when I first started learning Tai Chi, but I came to a greater understanding of their significance as time went on.

Attention and intention can be considered the yin and yang of the same coin, though each contains a dichotomy of its own. Attention has an active, yang aspect—as when one is listening to some sound—and a passive, yin aspect—as when

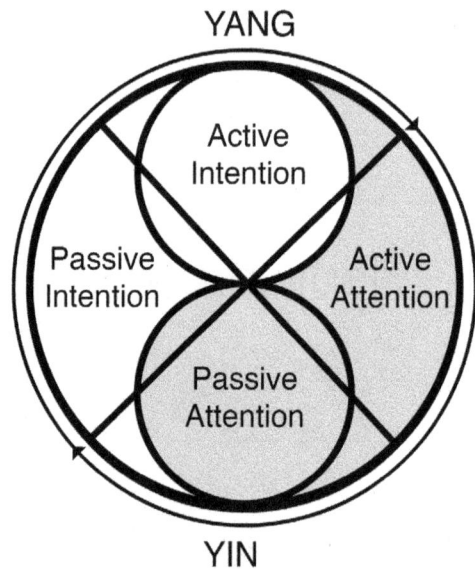

Figure 30.1 Both attention and intention have active, yang, aspects, and passive, yin, aspects.

one happens to catch drifts of sound on the wind. Intention's active, yang aspect, is the deliberate initiation of action—meaning to do something, such as reach out to pick up a glass of water—and its passive, yin aspect, is reaction—non-deliberate, instinctive response.

Note that non-deliberate does not mean or imply non- or unconscious. Mind and awareness are involved in all types of movement, just involved differently. Also, it is important to distinguish mind and attention from thought. Thought is something that goes on within the mind to which the mind frequently pays attention. But it doesn't have to, and the flow of thought can, with training, be ignored or suppressed, leaving awareness to observe sensation.

Attention (of both types) is associated with the autonomic, or sensory, nervous system, which transmits information from and about the world (including the state of one's body) to the mind. These nerves regulate yin chi flow within the body, and the chi field surrounding them flows from the extremities back into the Central Nervous System. In the limbs, the meridians for this inward flow lie within the outsides of the arms and the insides of the legs.[1]

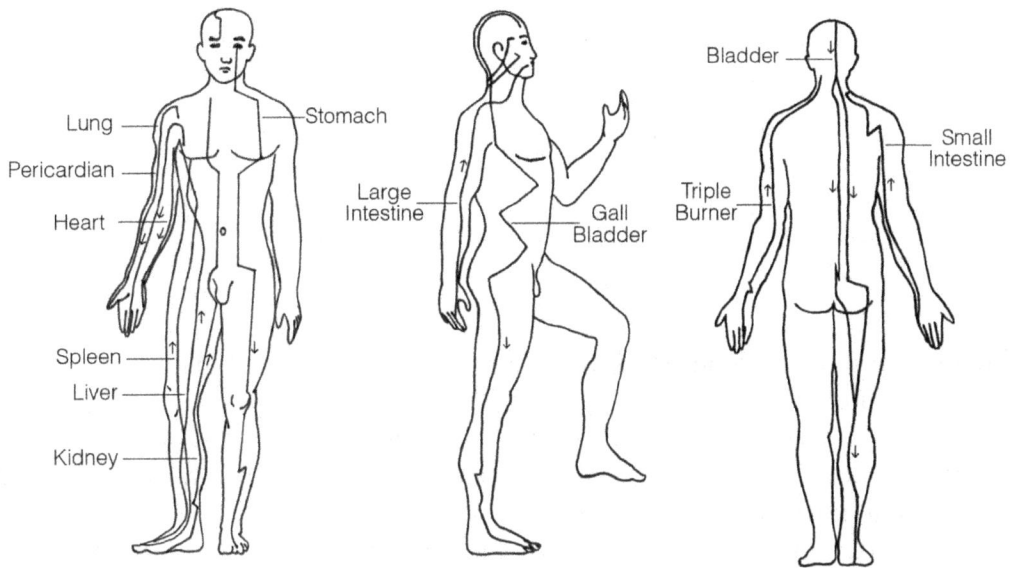

Figure 30.2 The Macrocosmic Orbit comprises the twelve major meridians that channel chi from the Microcosmic Orbit, through the torso, and into the limbs. The circuitry for the extremities consists of three meridians that channel chi into each limb and three that carry chi back into the Microcosmic Orbit.

Intention (of both types) is associated with the somatic nervous system, or the part of the nervous system that impels voluntary movement. These nerves regulate yang chi flow within the body, and the chi energy surrounding them flows from the Central Nervous System toward the extremities. In the limbs, the meridians for this outward flow lie within the insides of the arms and the outsides of the legs.

In each case, the yin aspect is simply the state of holding the nerve impulses in abeyance, and the yang aspect is the active sending or receiving of impulses. In all cases, it is the mind that regulates the way these two portions of the nervous system operate and handle the energy naturally flowing through them. The trick in Tai Chi is to eliminate thought from the process of movement and to use awareness to direct instinctual movement.

Tai Chi trains one to first use passive attention to sense the dynamic energy state that exists between the Tai Chi Chuanist and an opponent. When the opponent moves, the movement is felt on the physical level by the Tai Chi Chuanist's sensory apparatus, which consists of eyes, ears, nose, and skin. It also is felt on an energetic level that includes the chi field that surrounds the Tai Chi

Attention	Intention
Yin	Yang
Sensory input	Dynamic output
Active aspect: Focused	Active aspect: Deliberate movement
Passive aspect: Diffuse	Passive aspect: Instinctive movement
Autonomic nervous system	Somatic nervous system
Chi flows inward	Chi flows outward
Outsides of the arms & insides of legs	Insides of arms & outsides of legs

Chuanist's body. Information about the movement is then transmitted into his mind along the sensory nerves.

As soon as the dynamic energy state changes, it instantaneously transforms passive attention into active attention. This is the state of *wu wei*, or non-action, transforming, through action, into the yin/yang dichotomy of mutual interaction. The active attention triggers passive intention, which tends to produce instinctive reaction. But through Tai Chi's physical and mental training, that instinctive response is controlled and directed rather than haphazard, allowing the Tai Chi Chuanist to use active intention to push a wave of nerve impulses into a specific body part (yang usage) or to suck the energy back into himself (yin usage). Ideally, the resulting movement is of a type that seamlessly blends deliberate, purposeful action with the mindless speed of raw reaction.

When you watch people doing Tai Chi, often it is possible to distinguish those who can direct an inner force or purpose within the outer movement from those who, however accomplished in the completeness and flow of their forms, simply go through the motions.

Learning Tai Chi is like creating a vessel—the form—and then learning to fill that vessel with the fluid energy that we call chi. There are other exercises, notably chi kung, that can do the same thing, but Tai Chi's unique aspect is that it also trains the practitioner to mobilize the chi, both more powerfully through its natural circuits and more specifically into various body parts, in various ways, to lend practical utility to the chi and to the movements. This can be for martial purposes, but exercise and health are natural outcomes, even if one does not desire to engage in martial activity.

The movements of Tai Chi create physical alignments that are conducive to the propagation and channeling of wave energy—both physical and energetic, usually in tandem. One result of correct alignments of muscle, sinew, and bone is the ability to produce martial force. These same alignments also facilitate the production and accumulation of chi in the tantien, and they open up the major joints and muscles to eliminate blockages that inhibit the proper and strong flow of chi. They also give the practitioner, through specific techniques, a greater ability to control the flow of chi through the two major meridians that comprise the Microcosmic Orbit (Figure 30.3) and to direct it into the legs at the sacral plexus and into the arms at the brachial plexus (Figure 30.4). Active intent is a primary motivator of chi mobilization, the other primary motivator being the way one breathes. (See "Abdominal Breathing," previously.) Intent is the mental push that propels a pulse or wave of chi energy through the body by sending a mental sense of purpose down appropriate nerves.

Notice that this is not the same as deliberate movement, such as reaching out for a glass of water. In doing that, your mind has a desire or thought and instructs your muscles to act: I want water, it's over there, reach out for it. Movement caused by intention eliminates the step of the mind's deliberation. Instead, passive intent opens a clear pathway to an objective, and active intent immediately generates movement simply by intending it, without the extra steps taken by thought. In the case above, you feel thirst, and the next instant you are taking a sip of water.

The twin concepts of attention and intention are highlighted by two questions: Why do you practice Tai Chi, and how do you practice? Your reasons for

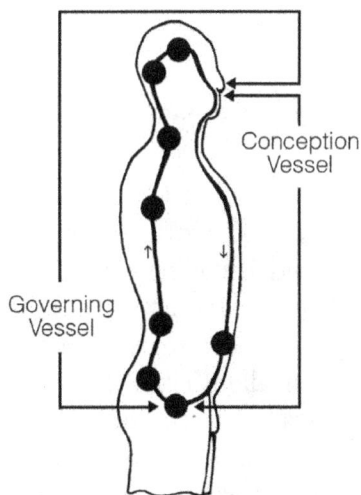

Figure 30.3 The Microcosmic Orbit consists of the body's two primary chi channels: the Conception Vessel and the Governing Vessel.

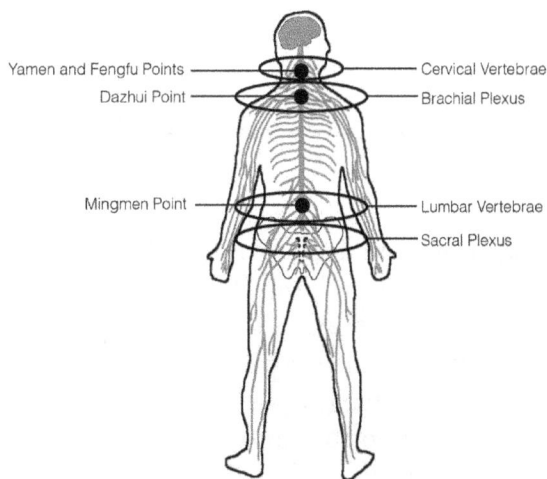

Figure 30.4 Important nerve plexus centers, spinal sections, and acupuncture points located along the Governing Vessel. Chi is channeled into the legs at the sacral plexus, and it is channeled into the arms at the brachial plexus.

Dualism

Dualism is defined as any system which implies a binary pattern, but which is characterized less by a complementary thesis and antithesis tending to resolve into a synthesis than by two opposed principles. The Manichean and Gnostic religions were moral dualisms. Some cosmic forms for division into two parts—such as the Chinese year split into two halves, one (Yang) in which the active and benign forces predominate, and the other (Yin) in which the passive and malign forces prevail—are binary systems rather than dualisms, because the double, contradictory aspects are synthesized within a system of wider scope. R. Bertrand, in *La Tradition secrète* (Paris 1943), speaking about this Yang–Yin symbol, observes: "The dualism of religion (or of mystic or cosmic philosophy) is theoretical and superficial; in actual fact, there is always something extra—a third term which prevents the two opposing terms from cancelling each other out, forcing both these force-principles to yield, that is, to function alternately and not simultaneously. Thus, the black and white of the Yin–Yang bounded by the circle of stability, t'ai-chi, combine to form in effect a ternary system, the Tao." However, this solution by means of the "third term" serves less to "resolve" the problem than to prolong it indefinitely since it encourages the persistence of the dualist state by virtue of the inner equilibrium which it implies. It is as if, in the symbolism of alchemy, the twin currents—ascending and descending—of solution and coagulation were kept in perpetual rotation. But this is in fact not the case: the positive forces triumph in the end—they transmute matter (that is, the passive, negative or inferior principle), redeem it and bear it upwards.

—J.E. Cirlot
A Dictionary of Symbols

practicing can be very important to the success of your practice. One excellent reason to practice is for health. There are a lot of ideas and stories about the health benefits of Tai Chi that may or may not be true, and I won't go into them here. But at its least, Tai Chi is a good, if not total, exercise, and as such, it has beneficial effects on physical health even without attention and intention. It promotes leg strength, stability, relaxation, correct structural alignments, flexibility, and body control, among others. All of these are critically important to good health—a claim with which I think almost every Tai Chi practitioner would agree. The other reasons for practicing Tai Chi will not so readily reach a consensus. They are self-development (spiritual advancement) and martial effectiveness.

Not always, but quite often, Tai Chi players will be drawn to the art for one of these reasons or the other, for Tai Chi contains a good bit of mystique with regards to both aspects. Tai Chi has always been billed as the soft and gentle

> The master of the mind is the mind-intent. The mind acts as only an assistant to the mind-intent. When the mind moves, it does so only because of the mind-intent; when the mind-intent arises the ch'i will follow.
>
> —Chen Kung
> Cultivating the Chi

martial art, the meditational martial art, the spiritual martial art. Consequently, it attracts a lot of people who are seeking spiritual advancement or mental and emotional comfort and release. Many of these people practice Tai Chi almost exclusively for the health, meditational, and self-development aspects, to the exclusion of the martial. When you watch these people practice, the movements are often beautiful and flowing, but sometimes they also seem devoid of content, of meaning. They seem empty, as if the players are waving their arms around in specific patterns without the intent or purpose. It is as if they have created an ornate container that holds nothing.

Tai Chi has a meditational, self-development aspect that is very important, but the art was originally developed to impart martial utility and as a way to increase and manipulate internal energy. Without intent or purpose, the movements are empty, and if empty, they cannot truly succeed in either their meditational purpose or their ability to enhance health and well-being. Certainly, an empty form cannot possibly magnify, store, propel, and channel internal energy.

Intention also is bound up in martial purpose and is inextricably tied to the question of how a particular movement or movements can be used in combat situations. I've met a lot of the exercise and meditational variety of Tai Chi players, and they all have some vague notion that Tai Chi is good for self-defense, and many have a belief that Tai Chi will come to their rescue in a time of crisis. That belief might not be well founded, because these individuals have not practiced Tai Chi with any sort of martial intent. Consequently, while their movements might basically go the right way, their body alignments and their internal energy aren't doing what they're supposed to do, and so the movements are ineffective for self-defense. Worse, because the alignments and energy channels aren't optimal, the movements are less effective for the meditational and spiritual aspects as well as for the health benefits that Tai Chi can impart.

My purpose here is not to disparage those who do not care for Tai Chi's martial aspect. Truthfully, I'm only a middling at the martial aspects myself, though I have practiced them some. For me, the feeling of the flow of energy is what is important. But I very much like the way that practicing Tai Chi's martial applications helps teach in a practical way the lessons of chi mobilization. What

I'm getting at is that, as far as I can tell, to make Tai Chi the truly effective and superior art it can be, the practice of it has to engage meaning that goes beyond the simple physical exercise and beyond the spiritual meditation. The practitioner must accept the intent and method of martial purpose because that is what develops the depth and range of both attention and intention within the practitioner, and those are what are used, to a large extent, to increase, drive, and manipulate the chi.

The reality is that to make Tai Chi truly effective on all levels—the physical, mental, emotional, and spiritual—it must be practiced with intent—as if one is really doing something. You must actually feel as though you are accomplishing a real task—even if you are doing it slowly and gently—and not just waving your arms and floating through the air. A lot of peaceful people who are attracted to Tai Chi for its positive physical and spiritual qualities might be turned off by the violence inherent in practicing it as a martial art, but, unfortunately, they are short-changing themselves by practicing the art as if it is all mystical form and no practical substance.

This doesn't mean that those of you who are not interested in Tai Chi's martial aspects must become martial artists. But it does mean that you have to learn at least a little bit about the martial purposes so that you can use that as a guide in learning to magnify, store, mobilize, and direct and focus your internal energy. The beauty of intention is that it is relatively easy to sense and to arouse. And from there, it's possible to delve more deeply into attention.

As you can see, attention and intention may be two sides of the same coin, but that coin can be spent in a number of different ways. As my karateka friend promised, Tai Chi does get better with age.

> That the warriors of old flocked to our peaceful hermitages to foster their martial skills is no paradox; they came to learn how to apply the secret of emptiness, how to ensure that the enemy's sword, though aimed at flesh, encounters void, and how to destroy the foe by striking with dispassion.
>
> —Taoist Abbot
> In John Blofeld
> *Taoist Mysteries and Magic*

31. Invest in Loss

The wisdom of the Tai Chi Classics leaves Tai Chi practitioners with a number of important ideas, principles, and practical advice. Among those is "Invest in loss." At first glance, the phrase itself might seem to be an oxymoron. After all, "investment" should accrue rather than diminish—though obviously not all investments pan out. But why would anybody deliberately put effort into losing? As usual, Tai Chi asks you to look beneath the surface.

The idea of investment is pretty straightforward. You put in capital—time, effort, money, and so forth—with the expectation of a reward over time. At its most basic in Tai Chi, investing in loss can indicate the expenditure of time and effort to learn the form and to continue to practice it. The loss is that half-hour to hour a day that you spend doing Tai Chi instead of something else. It's the loss of comfort reflected in the sore muscles and achy joints that sometimes accompany long-term physical practices. And it's understanding that the movements you've practiced diligently are never quite right and constantly have to be redone, adjusted, or realized in a different way.

In that context, I'm reminded of an anecdote about a great Tai Chi master. When asked if he'd ever done a perfect set of Tai Chi, he replied, "I thought I did last week, but this week, I did one even better." Despite the wryness of his reply, the meaning is clear: Even with his superior skill at Tai Chi, had he not continued to invest time and energy in his art—had he not continued to lose—he would not have continued to progress.

These sorts of investments are easy to see as a tangible quantities, and the results also are tangible: smoother, more flowing movements that are centered and grounded, producing a greater sense of physical capability and well-being. But other benefits that follow, while not exactly tangible, also are manifest. Through investment in daily practice, one experiences many sorts of loss that are really gains: loss of tension, loss of instability, and loss of improper body alignments.

Through investment in the meditational aspect of Tai Chi, one begins to divest oneself of erroneous, wayward, and careless thought. In a sense, Tai Chi asks you to "lose your mind," for the ultimate loss is loss (or at least suppression) of ego, or the mental desire to always

> It is not uncommon for accomplished students to lose the ability they had previously acquired to balance and coordinate the whole body when they concentrate on correcting specific mistakes pointed out within their posture. In this case, they lose awareness of their body "as a whole" as they focus only on fixing an individual part; for instance, the placement of a shoulder, hand, knee, or foot. The actual solution usually lies in adjusting a defect in the core or foundation of the student's posture and the other body parts generally will fall correctly into place.
>
> —William Ting
> *Essential Concepts of Tai Chi*

win or look good in the eyes of our fellow humans. Through this investment of calming the mind, we lose the need to observe ourselves from some theoretical outside perspective—a perspective that is filled with often erroneous suppositions of how others see us and what they think of us—and begin to observe ourselves from within.

In *Movements of Magic*, Bob Klein writes: "Letting go is a basic, if not the basic principle of T'ai-chi-Ch'uan."[1] In truth, investing in ego loss is one of the principal challenges of push hands practice, and it highlights another definition of "invest," which also means to give power or authority to, as in an investiture ceremony. In this meaning, you authorize, empower, and ordain someone or something to carry on with a given duty or procedure.

In push hands, you invest an opponent with the opportunity to invade your space and do something to you that most of us hate: push you around at close quarters. In other words, the loss is in allowing yourself to be pushed—to "lose" the fight. Fighting the pressure that your opponent puts on you is, itself, resistance to loss. Instead, one must learn that if resistance is met in one direction, then the accurate response is to lose (sink and turn) and then move in a different direction, seeking an emptiness in which there is no resistance—an emptiness in which re-

> No one ever profited from any undue benefit without paying for it in the form of unexpected or inexorable losses. Small benefits bring about small losses and big benefits big losses.
>
> —Cheng Man-ching
> *T'ai Chi Ch'uan*

sistance is lost, resulting in an investment in non-resistance that results in your opponent's loss.

Moreover, investing in loss is understanding that your efforts will not produce immediate results, either in practice of the form or in push hands. This is an important thing to keep in mind in our age of instant gratification. A Tai Chi buddy related a conversation he had with a young man who sincerely thought he was really good at kung fu because he could manipulate his game controller expertly during martial arts video games. Instant gratification and fanciful desires rarely produce genuine results. Instead, the mobility, energy, and skills imparted by the Tai Chi form accrue steadily over time in an almost imperceptible fashion, only revealing themselves after long periods of seemingly futile effort. And these long periods of apparent pointless work can definitely make one question the investment in one's practice, making it seem like wasted effort—a loss of the capital of time and effort.

"Invest in loss" is similar to a number of quotes by various people on the dichotomy of failure and success and how the latter follows only from the former. You might have your favorite; I'm choosing the following:

Failure is the key to success; each mistake teaches us something.
> —Morihei Ueshiba
> Founder of Aikido[2]

We learn wisdom from failure much more than from success. We often discover what will do by finding out what will not do; and probably he who never made a mistake never made a discovery.
> —Samuel Smiles
> Scottish author[3]

Nothing fails like success because we don't learn from it. We learn only from failure.
> —Kenneth Boulding
> Economist and systems scientist[4]

The idea is that one does not become expert at anything in an instant or without patient effort. One must repeatedly do things wrong before being able to funnel matters into a channel that is more correct. Growth results only from failure to move or behave properly and then trying again and again in different ways until something like success is approached. These failures are investments in loss that lead one farther along one's path.

Investing in loss—letting go—can serve as a rule for many aspects of life, such as marriage, work, play, and human interactions in the public sphere. Investing in loss can help eliminate destructive habits, erroneous thought, ungrounded expectations, or any of the other sundry elements of life that hold us back or otherwise prevent us from moving forward. It can do this simply by telling us that we can let go of the anchors that retard our progress and that we can navigate around blockages that impede us rather than futilely butting up against them.

Ultimately, though, no matter how diligently and determinedly we practice or how proficient we become, we will, in an instant, lose it all as we step through the door of death. We've all heard the adage about death and wealth that goes: You can't take it with you. But perhaps that statement isn't fully accurate. Certainly you can't take wealth or items with you, but if there is something beyond life and you can take some qualities with you, those would be aspects of personal development gained through life experiences, and personal development is fostered by investing in loss.

As in Tai Chi, investments in doing and in striving for accuracy and meaning in life are what are important, not achievements, per se, which will always be lost or superseded in the end. Perhaps the doing is enough.

It is certain that virtually all Taoist practice—yogic, philosophical, quietist and mystical—was based on experiencing the reconciliation of opposites, on conscious unification of the seemingly disparate and multiple, on direct perception of the identity of being and non-being, action, and non-action.

—John Blofeld
Taoist Mysteries and Magic

32. The Infinity Twist

The litany of important ideas to observe in Tai Chi is quite long. We have to pay attention to this and that and this other, all while we're doing thus and such and meditating on our movement and the non-movement within that movement. And trying to remember what comes next.

Phew!

We have to relax, drop our awareness of weight and energy into our legs—one at a time, clearly and distinctly. We have to move in a way that unfolds and refolds our bodies in specific patterns. We have to open and round the joints so that the energy can flow through them correctly. Moreover, we have to learn to do all this with as little muscular exertion as possible.

And importantly, we have to learn to spiral that energy from our torsos into the legs, where it rebounds from the feet and spirals back up into pelvic area, which includes the hips and waist. This is where the energy is redirected into the torso, which can be done in various ways. Those various ways, which are the different force/energy applications of Tai Chi as defined by the Four Cardinal Energies—Wardoff, Rollback, Press, and Push—are not the main subject of this article, though we might touch on them. Instead, we'll look at how a core secret of Tai Chi movement within the pelvic area can transform and direct the energy effectively. Why, in other words, "the waist is the commander," as is stated in the Tai Chi Classics, and why Tai Chi is called Tai Chi. I'll refer to this core movement as the Infinity Twist.

When those not in the know observe Tai Chi movements, they usually see the motions of the limbs—especially the arms. Those in the know understand that the real area of the body to observe is below the thorax: the waist, hips, and legs. All those arm movements are just being motivated by pulses or waves of combined motion and energy that originate in the lower body. (Figure 32.1) But it takes control to refine and manipulate those pulses into useful work. The old analogy from the Tai Chi Classics is: The legs are the people, the waist is the commander, and the arms and hands are the army or the state. The collective power of the people give strength and energy to the commander, who then directs his troops or, alternately, his government, into action.

Each of these three elements must be strong in order for the whole to function well. An excellent leader with a well-trained army will lose the war if his people do not support him with their strength; a weak leader causes a disjunction between the people and the government; and a dysfunctional military/government will leave the best of leaders at a disadvantage, even if he is backed by a strong populous. In the optimum situation, the people urge—and surge—and the commander, sensing that internal movement, directs his forces—army and government—appropriately. Or the people are quiet, and the leader and army remain quiescent.

Right in the middle of the Tai Chi dynamic is the commander—the waist—and here is where the raw force and energy from the legs, as expressed by the hips, are combined and directed into useful upper body movements. But the pelvic area, in and of itself, isn't the commander. It's just the house of the commander—where the commander has the physiological tools necessary to

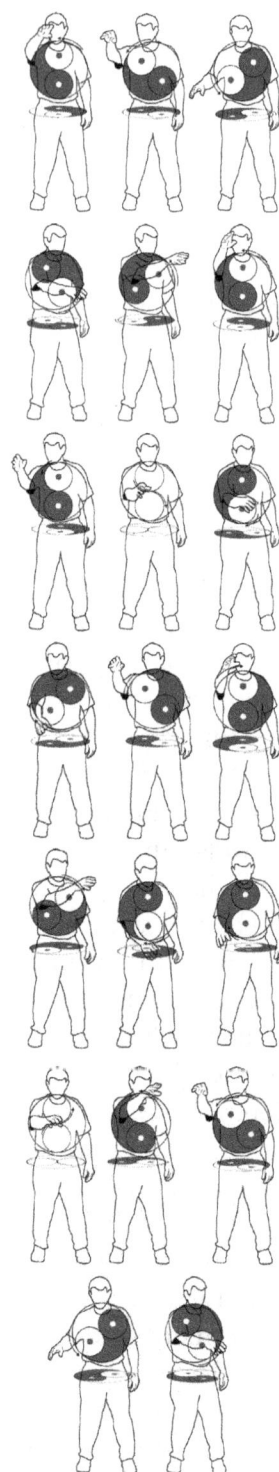

Figure 32.1 Chan-ssu Chin's most basic form winds the energy through a pattern that mimics the tai chi symbol. While the waist movements, propelled by alternate pushes from the legs, circle around the horizontal taiji-tu's circumference and then weave through its center, your loosely held arm simultaneously traces the same path on the vertical symbol.

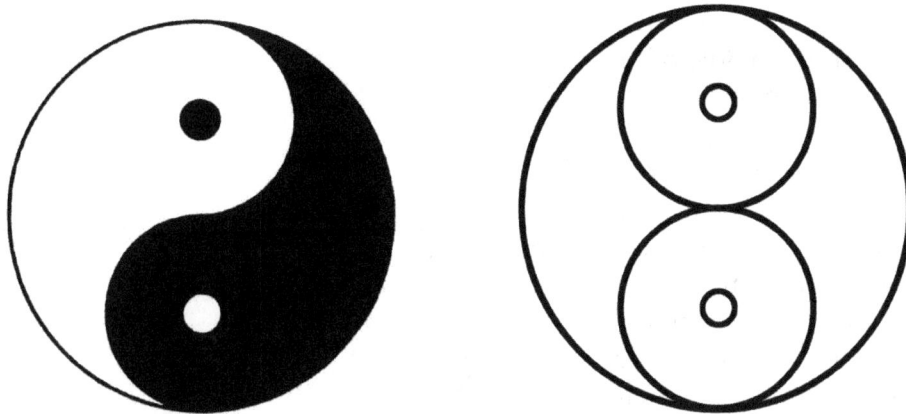

Figure 32.2 The tai chi symbol depicts the major forces of opposition and cooperation that underlie the functioning of reality. Left, it is depicted in its normal form, right, in its doubled form, which contains the Infinity Twist.

effect proper control, such as the hip joints, the flexible connection between the lumbar vertebra and the pelvis, and the ability to flex the *kua*, or the fold between the torso and upper thigh.

These tools are utilized by the true commander, which is the specific figure eight movement I'm calling the Infinity Twist. The shape of it is seen in the center of the doubled taijitu (Figure 32.2). It is a movement central to the large number of principles that the Tai Chi Chuanist must pay attention to because it is the core of Tai Chi's spiraling action and ability to store and release energy without losing momentum. It's not more important than sung, say, or maintaining certain body alignments, or other crucial principles of Tai Chi. It's equally important. You can't pick up something without your shoulder, arm, and hand working in conjunction. To effect correct movement, all the parts of the body that are involved must coordinate their efforts in accordance with correct principles. It is the same with the combined dynamics of the Infinity Twist, sung, and a handful of other important Tai Ch principles.

There are fascinating aspects about this core movement, for the Infinity Twist is active at the interface within the body where raw energy is refined and directed and where yin and yang movements and energies exchange and interchange. I've written a lot about the many syncretic aspects of the taijitu—the tai chi symbol—elsewhere in this book and in *Circling the Square: Observations on the Dynamics of Tai Chi Chuan*, so I'll try not to replicate much of that material here.

The Infinity Twist is the central fig-ure-eight in the middle of the taijitu. It's the infinity symbol. And, as that might indicate, it holds a whole lot more. It lies at the center of almost every Tai Chi movement, large and small, and that presence is the reason the art is named after the ideas exemplified by the tai chi symbol. To the point here, it is the way the Tai Chi exponent rotates his or her sense of movement, gravity, centered-ness of mass, and energy field in a fig-ure eight pattern around an axis.

The most important axis is Central Equilibrium, or an imaginary line dropped from the crown of your head, through your torso, through your per-ineum, and into the ground midway between your feet when you're standing in a normal front-facing stance. (Figure 32.3) In this case, the axis of Central Equilibrium stabs straight through the

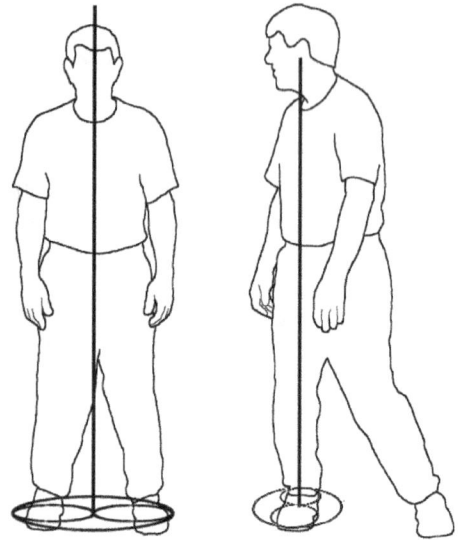

Figure 32.3 The Tai Chi exponent rotates his or her sense of movement, gravity, and cen-teredness of mass in a figure eight pattern around an axis.

crossing point where the two internal circles of the taijitu intersect. But there are two side axes, as well, and each can substitute for Central Equilibrium when one's weight is on one side or the other. Some Tai Chi movements emphasize Central Equilibrium, while others rely more on the side axes for single-weighted stability and release of power. Yet others transition through a combination of two or even all three axes during the movement.

In the early stages of a person's Tai Chi development, the Infinity Twist will be entirely absent in the novice's body. You can wave your arms around in Tai Chi movements all day long, but if they aren't connected through the move-ment of the waist to the energy of the legs, then those upper-body motions are empty. With long-term practice of the form, the twist eventually will appear. At first, it might be askew and wobbly, but with form practice come greater con-trol, and it will take on a smoother circulation.

This is because the twist is built into the movements of the form. Practiced regularly and correctly over a period of time, the movements of the form engrain the twist into the exponent's usual daily body movements. It often is said that Grasping Bird's Tail is the most important sequence of movements within the Tai

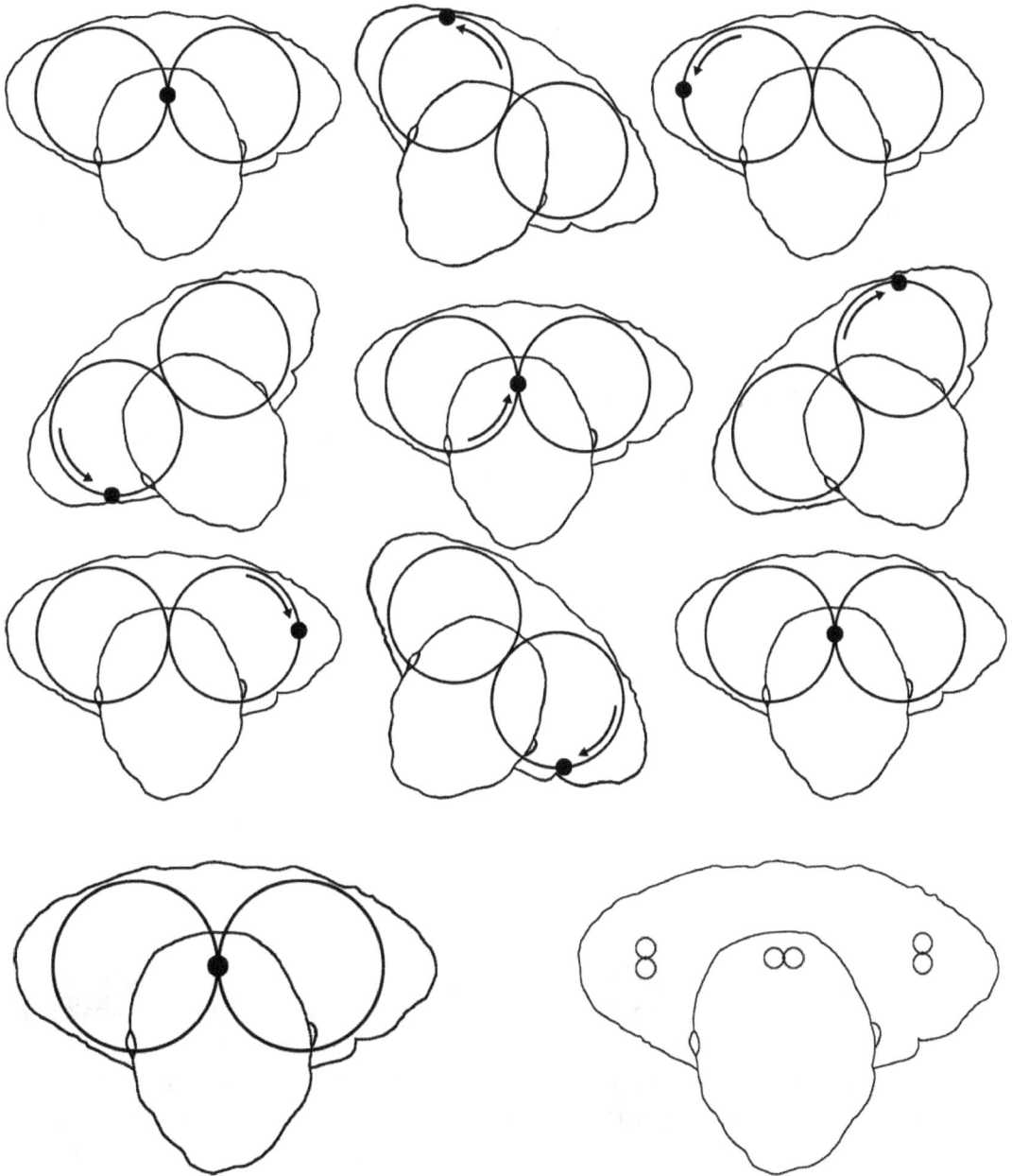

Figure 32.4 In the beginning, the size of the Infinity Twist is as large as it can be within the body, with the crossing point at Central Equilibrium and the far edges of the circles reaching to the outside edges of the hips. The movement is fairly large and easy to discern, and it generally remains so during normal daily form practice. But as time progresses, the practitioner gains the ability to severely reduce the diameter of the twist.

Chi form because all the secrets of the form are contained in this one cluster. On one level, this means that each of the Thirteen Postures is represented within this group, making Grasping Bird's Tail a mini-primer of basic Tai Chi postures. But perhaps more important, the Grasping Bird's Tail sequence contains and trains the Infinity Twist.

In the beginning, the size of the Infinity Twist is as large as it can be within the body, with the crossing point at Central Equilibrium and the far edges of the circles reaching to the outside edges of the hips. (Figure 32.4) The movement is fairly large and easy to discern, and it generally remains so during normal daily form practice. But as time progresses, the practitioner

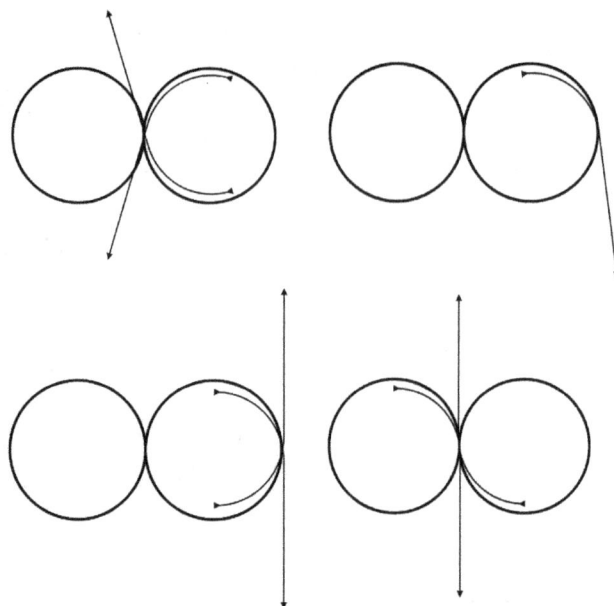

Figure 32.5 Wardoff (top left) is released diagonally through the curves in either direction. Rollback (top right) can be found in any of the curves that can be released tangentially away from the Infinity Twist. Press (bottom left) is released along the outer edges of either circle, either straight forward or straight back. And Push (bottom right) is released through the center, either straight forward or straight back. (Each diagram shows the forward and backward direction of movement only for the right side.)

gains the ability to severely reduce the diameter of the twist. The idea is to make the twist as small as possible inside the body, eventually becoming too small and hidden for the average person to perceive it. But it is there, centered on one of the three axes, and it remains just as powerful in its ability to circulate energy as it was when it was larger. Or perhaps even more so, since everything can happen so much more quickly and shockingly when energy is released from a small twist.

The Infinity Twist is what takes in energy, turns it into its opposite, and then releases it. And each of the four Cardinal Energies—Wardoff, Rollback, Press, and Push—are released by or find a home in, one section of the Infinity Twist, in both their yang and yin aspects—for fa jing or for neutralizing. Wardoff is released diagonally through the curves in either direction. Rollback can be found in any of the curves that can be released tangentially away from the Infinity Twist.

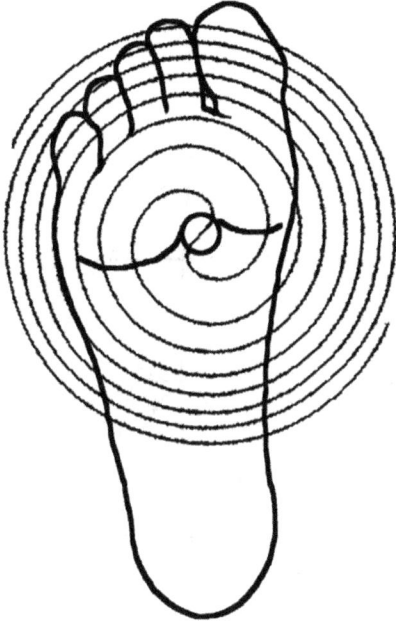

Figure 32.6 There is an infinity twist in the sole of the foot, centered on the Bubbling Well of the sole, that can spiral in and out in either direction.

Press is released along the outer side of either circle, either straight forward or straight back. And Push is released through the center, either straight forward or straight back. (Figure 32.5)

Because the energy spirals down the leg to the foot then changes direction in the foot and rebounds in a spiral that twists back up the leg in the opposite direction, there also is, in the sole of the foot, an Infinity Twist. This is the structure that smoothly transforms the downward spiral into the upward one, and its axis is the Bubbling Well. (Figure 32.6) The Infinity Twist in the sole is, of course, much smaller to begin with than the one in the waist, and another difference between the two is their orientation. In the waist, it is side to side, while in the foot, it is front-to-back. And like the Infinity Twist in the waist, the one in the sole also shrinks over time, becoming smaller and smaller, trying to approximate the infinitely tiny, at which time, it expands to take in the world.

The taijitu holds many of Tai Chi's more profound functional and philosophical principles in a simple yet infinitely fascinating symbol. The Infinity Twist is one of the most important and demonstrates that the art of Tai Chi truly deserves the name the Grand Ultimate, for it incorporates the principles of the very foundations of reality.

Elsewhere Lao-tzu says: I have three treasures which I guard and cherish. The first is compassion; the second frugality; the third spirit. Compassion begets courage; frugality begets a liberal spirit; humility begets supremacy. Courage without compassion, liberality without frugality, supremacy without humility—these spell death!"

—John Blofeld
Taoist Mysteries and Magic

Tai Chi's Structural Bows

Tai Chi Chuan's correct operations are dependent on the practitioner assuming a solid foundation. This usually is described as sung: feeling as if one is sitting, which positions one's body weight directly over the pelvis. In turn, this sitting allows all one's sense of weight and energy to settle downward into the lower abdomen (tantien) and legs.

But there is more to a solid foundation than just standing correctly or moving through the Tai Chi postures with correct physical stances. One also must sense the way that chi energy flows through the torso and limbs. This flow tends to be perceived mostly within the principal yang channels since those are the pathways that send energy forth rather than receive it. Over time, the sensations of these flows produce the feeling of having three curving, energetic structures within the body: Tai Chi's structural bows. The structural bows are not the same as the bow-and-arrow-like forces Tai Chi creates within the torso and limbs for storing and releasing energy. The structural bows are energetic in nature, while the bow-and-arrow forces are manipulations of the sinews.

One can most readily feel the structural bows when assuming the chi kung posture known as Standing Post. The primary bow is the leg bow—the arc from the feet through the legs and pelvis—because the legs are the body's foundation. If you don't create the leg bow first, you can't manifest the other two bows. The leg bow is created by utilizing the sitting posture and tucking the buttocks under slightly, making it seem like one is perched on a three-legged stool with the practitioner's legs forming two of the stool legs and the third leg being an imaginary extension of Central Equilibrium that runs from the pelvis to the floor.

The second most-important bow is the back bow, which runs along the spine. It requires, in addition, a slight tucking in of the chin, which straightens the cervical vertebrae, allowing the chi to flow unimpeded through the neck and head. Both the leg bow and the back bow can be created without bringing the arm bow into play, but the arm bow cannot be created without first aligning the leg and back bows. The arm bow arcs out from the back and through both shoulders and arms, and it can be considered to consist of two bows: one for each arm.

Once one can achieve a stance that incorporates and activates all the structural bows, one can then readily feel how even minute pulses of energy from the legs can be transmitted through the composite bow structure to activate the limbs.

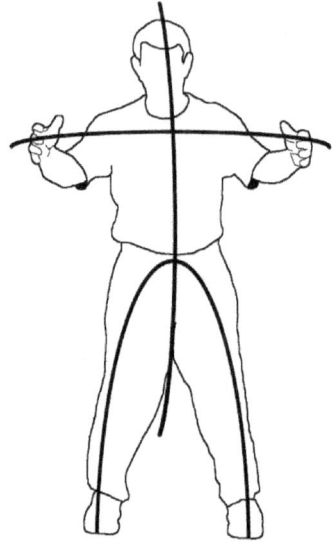

Conclusion

Tai Chi Chuan, whose movements constantly evoke the form of the taijitu—and thus the Golden Spiral—and embody profound interconnections with reality at large, carries deep and manifold universal meanings. Properly attended to, the art can assist one in transforming not only ill health into well-being and weakness into strength, but flat thinking into dimensional thinking. It's no wonder that Tai Chi is generally considered to be the most elegant as well as one of the most functional and effective of the martial arts—and one of the deepest philosophically. Thanks for joining me on this journey as I explored some of the possibilities of this timeless art. May your practice, whatever its purposes, bring you great benefits.

Moment

In the spread of the bird's tail
There is a moment like the warrior's
Dance of ten thousand tears.
The march must continue.
The winds of change....

Notes

Part I: Roots

A Historical and Personal Perspective on Tai Chi Chuan

1 "Zhang Sanfeng." *Wikipedia*, https://en.wikipedia.org/wiki/Zhang_Sanfeng.

Chang San-feng: His Life and Deeds

1 Gilbey, John F. (Robert W. Smith), *The Way of the Warrior* (North Atlantic Books, 1986).

Part II: Miscellaneous Matters

Christianity versus Chi

1 "Chinese Wand Exercise." *Wikipedia*, http://en.wikipedia.org/wiki/Chinese_Wand_ Exercise.
2 "Vicar bans anti-Christian exercise class Tai Chi from church hall." *Daily Mail*, http://www.dailymail.co.uk/news/article-1258888/Vicar-bans-anti-Christian- exercise-class-Tai-Chi-church-hall.html.
3 "Is the idea of chi compatible with the Christian faith?" *Got Questions*, http:// www. gotquestions.org/chi-Christian.html.
4 "Should a Christian Practice the Martial Arts?" http://www.equip.org/article/ should- a-christian-practice-the-martial-arts/

5 "Why Tai Chi and Catholicism Don't Mix." *Women of Grace*, http://www.-womenof- grace.com/blog/?p=338.

6 "Tai chi: occult, dangerous and not for Christians—we answer our critics." *The Free Press*, http://www.thefreepressonline.co.uk/news/1/2522.htm.

7 "Yoga and Christianity: Are They Compatible?—A Biblical Worldview Perspective." http://www.probe.org/yoga-and-christianity-are-they-compatible/.

8 "Christians and Kundalini." http://yogadangers.com/christianity-and-kundalini/.

9 Kundalini Energy and Christian Spirituality—Discussion." http://innerexplorations. com/ewtext/ke.htm.

10 "More on Kundalini Energy and Christian Spirituality, Including an Interview with Philip St. Romain." http://www.innerexplorations.com/ewtext/moreon.htm.

11 "Fatwa No: 252025—Ruling on practicing Tai Chi." http://www.islamweb.net/emainpage/index.php?page=showfatwa&Option=FatwaId&Id=252025.

12 "My Story: An experience of Jinn Possession." http://www.thejinn.net/chi_jinn_ my_story.htm.

13 "The Truth about Spontaneous Chi Kung (Jinns/Demonic Possession)." http:// www.dangerofchi.org/. (Note: This page opens with a veritable catalog of articles and resources for those who fear and demonize spiritual energies, the practices that foster them, and the cultures and religions that acknowledge these energies and their beneficial aspects.)

The Alchemy of Chi

1 Gershon, Michael D., MD, *The Second Brain: A Groundbreaking New Understanding of Nervous Disorders of the Stomach and Intestines* (Quill, 1998), p. 83.

Part III: Tai Chi that Isn't Tai Chi but Is Tai Chi

Introduction

1 Ting, William, *Essential Concepts of Tai Chi: It is - It is Not - IT IS* (Xlibris, 2015).
2 "Drawing Hands," M. C. Escher

The Twist

1 "The Twist." *Wikipedia*, https://en.wikipedia.org/wiki/Twist_(dance).
2 Stearns, Jean, and Stearns, Marshall Winslow, *Jazz Dance* (Da Capo, 1994).

AirDancers

1 *Bing Images*, http://www.bing.com/images/search?q=inflatable+sign+images&view =detailv2&&id=6C500A992243CF0C02952-FA3378B8B1E9205595B&selectedIndex=22&ccid=KTNYe5wa&simid=608046935219506489&thid=OIP.M29335 87b9c1af2559b7f4ffaa5172dd3o0&ajaxhist=0.

Tai Chi in the Driveway

1 *Bing Images*: http://www.bing.com/images/search?view=detailV2&ccid=Y49ChwPc &id=03EB-D87482197F56394E02B55DD3AA1068802AD7&q=u-joint&simid =608021680915615519&selectedIndex=2&ajaxhist=0.

2 *Bing Images*: http://www.bing.com/images/search?view=detailV2&ccid=SUhK3if%2b&id=02C03124E96447342060A2910671D97A9C1B21AC&q=differential&s imid=608045457834050083&selectedIndex=14&ajaxhist=0.

Part IV: Natural Patterns

Lemniscate

1 "Lemniscate." *Wikipedia*, https://en.wikipedia.org/wiki/Lemniscate.

2 *Taijitu Magazine*, http://www.phosphenepublishing.com/taijitumagazine.

3 "Spiric Section." *Wikipedia*, https://en.wikipedia.org/wiki/Spiric_section.

4 "Lemniscate." *Wikipedia*, https://en.wikipedia.org/wiki/Lemniscate.

5 "Torus." *Wikipedia*, https://en.wikipedia.org/wiki/Torus.

6 "Torus." *Wikipedia*, https://en.wikipedia.org/wiki/Torus.

7 "Cassini Oval." *Wikipedia*, https://en.wikipedia.org/wiki/Cassini_oval.

8 "Torus." *Wikipedia*, https://en.wikipedia.org/wiki/Torus.

9 "Torus." *Wikipedia*, https://en.wikipedia.org/wiki/Torus.

10 "Möbius Strip." *Wikipedia*, https://en.wikipedia.org/wiki/M%C3%B6bius_strip.

11 *Bing Images*, http://www.bing.com/images/search?view=detailV2&ccid=tqpcK% 2fBz&id=1400470BAD-D7A0C90692034F07CADB23F0929029&q=m.c.escher&simid=608014461074738359&selectedIndex=184&ajaxhist=0.

Spiral

1 "Archimedean spiral." *Wikipedia*, https://en.wikipedia.org/wiki/Archimedean_spiral.

2 "Golden Ratio." *Wikipedia*, http://en.wikipedia.org/wiki/Golden_ratio.

3 Zeising, Adolf, *Neue Lehre van den Proportionen des meschlischen Körpers* (1854), preface, from *Wikipedia* entry, "Golden ratio," http://en.wikipedia.org/wiki/Golden_ratio.

4 "Archimedean spiral." *Wikipedia*, https://en.wikipedia.org/wiki/Archimedean_spiral.

5 "Archimedean spiral." *Wikipedia*, https://en.wikipedia.org/wiki/Archimedean_spiral.

6 "Fermat's spiral." *Wikipedia*, https://en.wikipedia.org/wiki/Fermat%27s_spiral.

7 "Archimedes screw." *Wikipedia*, https://en.wikipedia.org/wiki/Archimedes%27_screw.

8 "Archimedes screw." *Wikipedia*, https://en.wikipedia.org/wiki/Archimedes%27_screw.

9 "Archimedes screw." *Wikipedia*, https://en.wikipedia.org/wiki/Archimedes%27_screw.

10 "Logarithmic spiral." *Wikipedia*, https://en.wikipedia.org/wiki/Logarithmic_spiral.

11 "Logarithmic spiral." *Wikipedia*, https://en.wikipedia.org/wiki/Logarithmic_spiral.

12 "Euler spiral." *Wikipedia*, https://en.wikipedia.org/wiki/Euler_spiral.

13 "Lituus." *Wikipedia*, https://en.wikipedia.org/wiki/Lituus_(mathematics).

14 "Hyperbolic spiral." *Wikipedia*, https://en.wikipedia.org/wiki/Hyperbolic_spiral.

15 "Poinsot spirals." *Wikipedia*, https://en.wikipedia.org/wiki/Poinsot%27s_spirals.

Curve

1 "Viviani's Curve." *Wikipedia*, https://en.wikipedia.org/wiki/Viviani%27s_curve.

2 "Lemniscate." *Wikipedia*, https://en.wikipedia.org/wiki/Lemniscate.

3 "Watt's curve." *Wikipedia*, https://en.wikipedia.org/wiki/Watt%27s_curve.

4 "Watt's linkage." *Wikipedia*, https://en.wikipedia.org/wiki/Watt%27s_linkage.

5 *Bing Images*, http://www.bing.com/images/search?view=detailV2&ccid=Pd%2f2zP qJ&id=F0FDBF9BECEEB-B277C04913366E7475EAEC606EF&q=Do+Nothing+Machine&simid=608029630892803234&selectedIndex=162&ajaxhist=0.

6 "Trammel of Archimedes." *Wikipedia*, https://en.wikipedia.org/wiki/Trammel_of_ Archimedes.

Doppler Style Tai Chi

1 "Longitudinal wave." *Wikipedia*, https://en.wikipedia.org/wiki/Longitudinal_wave.
2 https://upload.wikimedia.org/wikipedia/commons/thumb/9/9e/Doppler_effect.svg/768px-Doppler_effect.svg.png
3 http://i.ytimg.com/vi/fjaPGkOX-wo/maxresdefault.jpg

Under the Tai Chi Lens

1 Needham, Joseph, *Science and Civilization in China*, vol. IV, part 1: "Physics and Physical Technology," p. 82.
2 "Lens (optics)." *Wikipedia*, https://en.wikipedia.org/wiki/Lens_(optics).
3 "Lens (optics)." *Wikipedia*, https://en.wikipedia.org/wiki/Lens_(optics).
4 "Lens (optics)." *Wikipedia*, https://en.wikipedia.org/wiki/Lens_(optics).
5 "Camera obscura." *Wikipedia*, https://en.wikipedia.org/wiki/Camera_obscura.

Part V: Toying with Tai Chi

Tops and Gyroscopes

1 Top images:

Hand-thrown top: *Bing Images*, http://www.bing.com/images/search?q=Wooden+Toy+Tops&view=detailv2&&id=FD4AA757F-B2D0AA43ECD7F79D175DCEB5C1A3481&selectedIndex=135&ccid=uLD86VFT&simid=607994004044646251&thid=OIP.Mb8b0fce95153553df11815079e3b4b76o0&ajaxhis t=0.

Spindle top: *Bing Images*, http://www.bing.com/images/search?q=Wooden+Toy+ Tops&view=detailv2&&id=D064208FFAB-B9BE924FC09E8EE20AB4DB1D69E6E&selectedIndex=4&ccid=jz%2f2RxMV&simid=608020727328672 253&thid=OIP.M8f3ff647131563e57fcd324a91091271o0&ajaxhist=0.

Device-activated top: *Bing Images*, http://www.bing.com/images/search?q=Wooden+Toy+Tops&view=detailv2&&id=D622A35DAF092D11091A70C4A60F62F31E366852&selectedIndex=1&ccid=ACV%2fPqE6&simid=607988261665770354&thid=OIP.M00257f3ea13ab1ee3b39f66693b0a3f6H0&ajaxhist=0.

Mechanical top: *Bing Images*, http://www.bing.com/images/search?q=Vintage+Sp inning+Tops&view=detailv2&&id=AAE5083F9712D223FE0AAC12A39E3 5E6BE994AF0&selectedIndex=10&ccid=OXKE6Dmr&simid=6080311469 14873397&thid=OIP.M397284e839ab0fc00d509307c7281044o0&ajaxhist =0.

2 "Gyroscope." *Wikipedia*, https://en.wikipedia.org/wiki/Gyroscope.

3 *Bing Images*, https://www.bing.com/images/search?q=gyroscope&view=detail-v2& &id=88A50ED5256F4FBC8656013D868BDA5F7A214DB0&selected-Index=0 &ccid=yVWyzwnY&simid=608034514176311815&thid=OIP.M-c955b2cf09d87 0764fc6432516f3bf5bH0&ajaxhist=0.

Rubber Band

1 *Bing Images*, http://www.bing.com/images/search? view=detailV2&ccid=d3%2fkIS cH&id=5D8026999D3F6BF4AAACF44F3BA3F5744E39506D&q=rubber+b an d+airplane&simid=608037653881098000&selectedIndex=62&ajaxhist=0.

Magnet

1 *Bing Images*, http://www.bing.com/images/search?view=detailV2&ccid=tMI-UukO A&id=B2AF5062291E4DB824BE26E33039D1898A681A1C&q=Mag-netic+For ce&simid=608031361766263829&selectedIndex=5&ajaxhist=0.

Newton's Cradle

1 "Newton's Cradle." *Wikipedia*, https://en.wikipedia.org/wiki/ Newton%27s_cradle.

Magnets

1 *Bing Images*, http://www.bing.com/images/search?view=detailV2&ccid=tMI-UukO A&id=B2AF5062291E4DB824BE26E33039D1898A681A1C&q=Mag-netic+For ce&simid=608031361766263829&selectedIndex=5&ajaxhist=0.

Newton's Cradle

1 "Newton's cradle." *Wikipedia*, https://en.wikipedia.org/wiki/ Newton%27s_cradle.

Crack the Whip

1 "Snap the Whip." *Wikipedia*: https://en.wikipedia.org/wiki/Snap_the_Whip. Part VI: Principles and Operations

Attention and Intention

1 See my books, *The Wellspring: An Inquiry into the Nature of Chi* and *Circling the Square: Observations on the Dynamics of Tai Chi Chuan,* for more thorough discussions on the nature, generation, and mobilization of chi.

Invest in Loss

1 Klein, Bob, *Movements of Magic: The Spirit of T'ai-chi-Ch'uan* (Newcastle Publishing Co., 1984), p. 16.
2 *Brainy Quote,* http://www.brainyquote.com/quotes/quotes/m/moriheiues183597. html.
3 *Dangerously Irrelevant,* http://dangerouslyirrelevant.org/2008/07/we-learn-from-f. html.
4 *Dangerously Irrelevant,* http://dangerouslyirrelevant.org/2008/07/we-learn-from-f. html.

Phosphene Publishing Company

Publishes books and DVDs relating to fiction, literature, history, the paranormal, film, spirituality, and the martial arts.

For other great titles, visit
phosphenepublishing.com

www.ingramcontent.com/pod-product-compliance
Lightning Source LLC
Chambersburg PA
CBHW081150270326
41930CB00014B/3102